KETTLEBELL
TRAINING
FOR
STRENGTH AND POWER

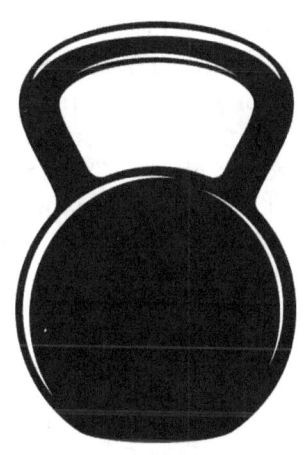

by

DAVE BELLOMO

ISBN-13: 978-1500176228
ISBN-10: 1500176222

This book is dedicated to my loving wife, Kelley, and our five beautiful children, Olivia, Victoria, Gabrielle, Peter, and Nicholas, without whose patience and support this work would have been impossible.

ACKNOWLEDGEMENTS

As always, thank you to my mentors Mike Murray, Tom Connolly, and Lanny Reed without whom strength training and physical culture would not be such a large part of my life. Thank you to Rik Brown of Liberty Strength Training and Louie Simmons of Westside Barbell for your great strength training insight and to Bill Hinbern of Superstrengthtraining.com for your wealth of Iron Game knowledge. A very special thanks to my editor, Andrew Ciotola, for the wonderful organization and layout of this book. Lastly, thanks to my clients and friends who continue to believe in me even after all of these years of early morning workouts and human guinea-pig sessions.

This book is for educational purposes. It is not intended as a substitute for individual health and fitness advice. Any use of the information contained in this book is at the discretion of the reader. The author disclaims any and all liability arising directly or indirectly from the use or application of any information contained in this book.

FOREWORD

KETTLEBELL TRAINING, REVISITED

Those of us who have been involved in strength training for the last few decades can well remember a time when kettlebells were nearly nonexistent in America. Today, kettlebells of various weights and shapes are a fixture in gyms across the country and the world. They are touted by some as the tool of choice for building up and slimming down, for men and women alike.

But as with any tool, kettlebells must be used intelligently for maximum results. David Bellomo is a seasoned veteran instructor with twenty-one years of experience in kettlebell, barbell, dumbbell, and bodyweight training. He has watched the growth of kettlebells from little more than a novelty to the cottage industry they are today. His view is not just that of a spectator on the sidelines or even a trainee. As one of the very first to distribute valuable how-to training information for correct and practical kettlebell usage, he was an integral part of their growth. Dave's fifteen years as a competitive power-lifter and thirty-one years in the strength training field are clearly evident in his presentation of kettlebell usage and practice.

I'm happy to announce today that my good friend Coach Bellomo is making his improved training methods available, once again, to those neophytes who wish to get started correctly to avoid bad habits as well as potential injury. Seasoned practitioners can expect some surprises for tweaking their form or picking up a valuable tip here and there. One thing is for sure: the methods found in this training manual present tried and true exercises and routines for everyone, male or female, of all ages, at every level of experience.

I highly recommend this long awaited training manual for anyone who wishes to use the kettlebell for total body strength and overall physical development.

Bill Hinbern
Super Strength Training
www.superstrengthtraining.com

TABLE OF CONTENTS

Single Clean: Russian Style
Alternating Clean
Single Outside Clean
Double Outside Clean

CHAPTER 4: SNATCH: THE UNDISPUTED KING OF KETTLEBELL LIFTS 48

Single Snatch
Double Snatch
Alternating Snatches

CHAPTER 5: OVERHEAD PRESS, PUSH-PRESS, AND JERK VARIATIONS 54

Two-Handed Overhead Press
Single Overhead Press
Double Overhead Press
Alternating Overhead Press
One-Stays-Up Overhead Press
Single & Double Bottoms-Up Press
Push Press & Jerk Variations

CHAPTER 6: BENT-OVER ROW VARIATIONS 64

Single Row
Double Row
Alternating Row
One-Stays-Up Row

CHAPTER 7: FLOOR PRESS VARIATIONS 69

Two-Handed Floor Press
Single Floor Press
Double Floor Press

Alternating (Seesaw) Floor Press
One-Stays-Up Floor Press

Side Bend (Windmill)
Squat Press
Sidewinder
Bent Press
Two-Hands Anyhow

Thick Bar Deadlift, Prone and Staggered Grips
Weighted Chin-Ups
Close-Grip Bench Press
Box Squats

Program Design
Power Days
Maximum Strength Days
Three-Day Program Sample
Four-Day Program Sample
Bonus Workouts
Mace / Hammer Swings, Chops & Twists
Stone Lifting and Throwing
Sandbags
Wheelbarrows, Sleds & Other Odd Objects

PREFACE

When I began writing this book, my intention was to compile a comprehensive guide for the development of kettlebell training programs. My hope was to illustrate how basic organizational phases could be manipulated to produce specific adaptations, using kettlebells as the primary strength-training implement. Simply put, my desire was to teach how organizing your training plan would produce better results. As I spent more time writing and speaking about the project with other strength professionals, I soon realized that my subject matter was too involved for a single book, that such a book would be too diluted to be of value and too long to be practical.

There are many "how-to" kettlebell manuals on the market, touting a bazillion exercises and workouts. Some are good; others are not. What appears to be lacking, however, is a guide that focuses on us-

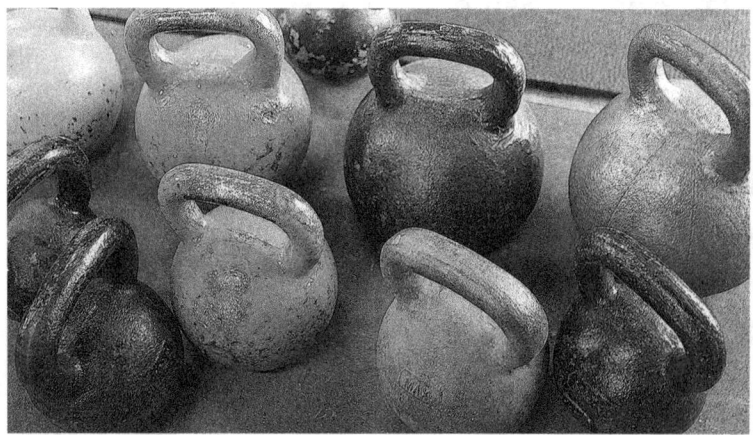

ing kettlebells specifically for developing strength and power rather than for conditioning, on which most books on this topic seem to focus. Many guides show shredded twenty-year-olds contorting their bodies with 35-pound bells, or performing hundreds of snatches with light weights. I am not discounting these practices if they are consistent with your training goals. I simply desire to fill the void in strength training regarding how kettlebells relate to true strength and power, and to show that there is a time for heavy, near maximal efforts, and that there is a time for explosive, power training.

In this book I wanted to explore such issues as modification of weight distribution during the descent of near maximal kettlebell snatches, or proper foot positioning for heavy, one-handed kettlebell presses. I will discuss the most successful formula I have found for program design, which might save you the trouble of repeating my mistakes. In response to requests from many clients and students, I will also touch on incorporating other training tools, such as hammers, dumbbells, barbells, and odd implements such as stones, sandbags, and thick bars. As we all know, the devil is in the details. Many books on the market list an endless number of exercises, but lack any real depth of information, causing beginners to scratch their heads and advanced lifters to wonder why they wasted their money. What I hope separates this work from the others is my attention to the finer points of program design and strength training technique. I want to show not only that kettlebells are outstanding training tools, but also how they can compliment other training implements to produce optimal results. I plan on accomplishing this by teaching you my personal methods for developing whole-body strength and power, methods that will carry over into all areas of your life. My hope is that you will learn at least one thing, make one minor change in your training, or glean one bit of knowledge that opens up new possibilities, so that the field of strength training moves forward, benefitting us all.

INTRODUCTION

A BRIEF HISTORY

Kettlebells and similar training weights have been around for millennia, though there are conflicting accounts of their exact time and place of origin. Popular belief holds that kettlebells are a Russian creation, stemming from the Russian kettlebell sport Girevoy, where lifters called "girevicks" use kettlebells called "gyra." In fact, they may have originated elsewhere. Stone weights resembling kettlebells have been found in Greece, where early Olympians may have used them in training. The Russian word "gyra" may be of Persian origin and closely resembles the Persian words "hera" and "gera" in pronunciation, both of which translate to "weight".

The modern form of the metal kettlebell was likely created in the early 1600's. According to strength historian Bill Hinbern, these first modern kettlebells were used to weigh grain or other farm produce. Hinbern speculates that farmers and blacksmiths would fill downtime by playing catch with these early weights. They would swing and flip the kettlebells, usually weighing approximately 12 to 16 kg (26–35 lbs), to their partners. The partners would increase their distance from one another until someone missed, in which case the other partner was declared the winner. According to some sources, Russian soldiers of the period utilized this type of weight to develop strength for lifting cannonballs during wartime.

By the late 1800's, kettlebells were being used by the performing strongmen who traveled with circuses throughout Europe, North America, and parts of Asia. Famous strongmen such as Saxon, Sandow, Goerner, and Kryloff used kettlebells as main implements in their performances, though they likely used them more for shows and stunts than for training. Kettlebell training during this period was usually restricted to dif-

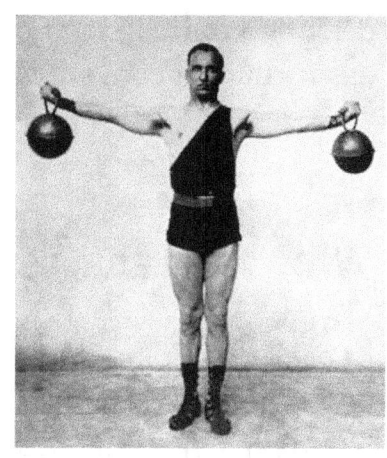

ferent types of swings, one- and two-handed flips, juggling, and pressing. Kettlebells might also appear in movements like the "Two-Hands Anyhow," sometimes in conjunction with dumbbells and barbells, where both hands were used to lift multiple heavy weights in a somewhat awkward fashion to a fully extended position overhead.

Girevoy, the Russian sport mentioned above, was created in the 1980's. Sport kettlebell competitions are usually organized into the biathlon or the long cycle categories. In biathlon, athletes perform

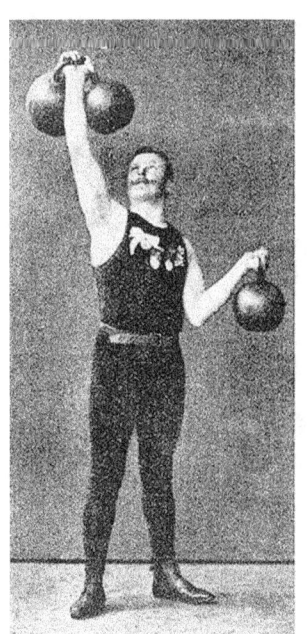

kettlebell jerks for ten minutes followed by snatches for ten minutes. In long cycle, athletes perform clean-and-jerks for ten minutes. The competitions have steadily increased in popularity in the last decade and can be found all over the world.

Kettlebells are also a staple training tool for organizations such as Crossfit, a varied, high-intensity training program designed to prepare people for any physical challenge they may face. In recent years martial artists have revived kettlebell training by using them extensively in rigorous conditioning programs designed to build strength and stamina without adding the unnecessary bulk of conventional bodybuilding programs.

WHY KETTLEBELLS?

Kettlebell training is arguably the most effective and efficient form of strength training ever created. It is based upon whole-body, real-life movements that today's fitness experts would call "functional," as opposed to muscle-group-specific styles of strength-training like bodybuilding. Fitness machines typically work in only one plane of movement, such as forward and backward or side-to-side. Many kettlebell exercises, however, incorporate movement into more than one plane, just as people move in real life. Some kettlebell exercises can be performed in a slow, controlled manner, while others must be performed in a more abrupt, "explosive" manner. They can be used to isolate a single muscle group, as well as for big, whole-

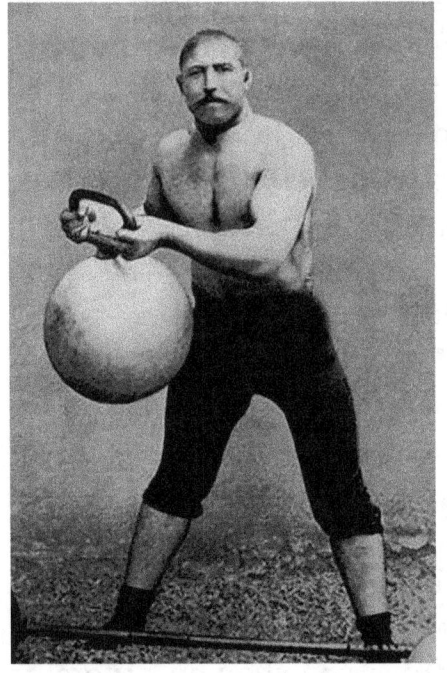

body movements. Kettlebells are not only versatile but also extremely durable, cost-effective, and space efficient.

While a dumbbell's weight is distributed symmetrically on either side of its central handle, a kettlebell's weight is one solid mass. This fact, as well as the increased distance of the kettlebell's center of mass from the lifter, means greater power is needed to perform many exercises than for a dumbbell of the same weight. This also makes the kettlebell ideal for performing ballistic, whole-body exercises such as cleans, snatches, and their variations. Kettlebells can be used either individually or in pairs. Kettlebells are more user-friendly than dumbbells in performing movements such as the high-pull, because the wide handle allows for comfort and correct body positioning. These Old-World weights are not just for the elite strongmen seen on television. Anyone who is healthy enough to strength-train can learn to use kettlebells. Whether you are a great athlete or a great-grandmother, these simple tools will help you to produce extraordinary results.

HEAVY KETTLEBELLS AND FEATS OF STRENGTH

Heavy kettlebells first received widespread attention in the heyday of the circus strongmen in the late 1800's. Arthur Saxon was reported to clean-and-press a 112-pound kettlebell while holding a 336-pound barbell in his other hand; bringing his Two-Hands Anyhow lift to 448 pounds. His bodyweight was approximately 200 pounds. Herman Goerner, another strength legend and a giant for his day, weighing in at a whopping 315 pounds, performed one-handed flips with a 171-pound kettlebell. Modern day Canadian strongman John Hadzi has exceeded this feat by flip-catching a 180-pound kettlebell with one hand, using a kettlebell with a considerably thicker handle than Goerner's. Hadzi also routinely performs multiple flips in a single throw with a 100+ pound kettlebell, also with one hand. Even the late, great World's Strongest Man competitor Jesse Marunde trained with heavy kettlebells, performing one-handed high pulls. (His hands were so large that they would not both fit on the handle.) Although nothing seemed heavy to Jesse, he credited heavy, 130+ pound kettlebell training for not only improving his loading times but also his ability to lift heavier stones.

So, what is the point? Why bother with such heavy kettlebells? What is the benefit of performing the low (1-3) rep sets that these weights sometimes demand? Heavy kettlebells test our grip, develop our whole-body strength, and push our limits. They make us pull, push and twist with everything we've got, lighting up our nervous systems like a fireworks display. Heavy kettlebells develop tendon and ligament strength like nothing else. If it is power you seek, heavy kettlebells are certainly the answer. They will build incredible explosive strength. Whether your goal is to hoist a limit lift, add repetitions to a low rep set, or move with the power of a superhero, you too can make tremendous progress with heavy kettlebell training.

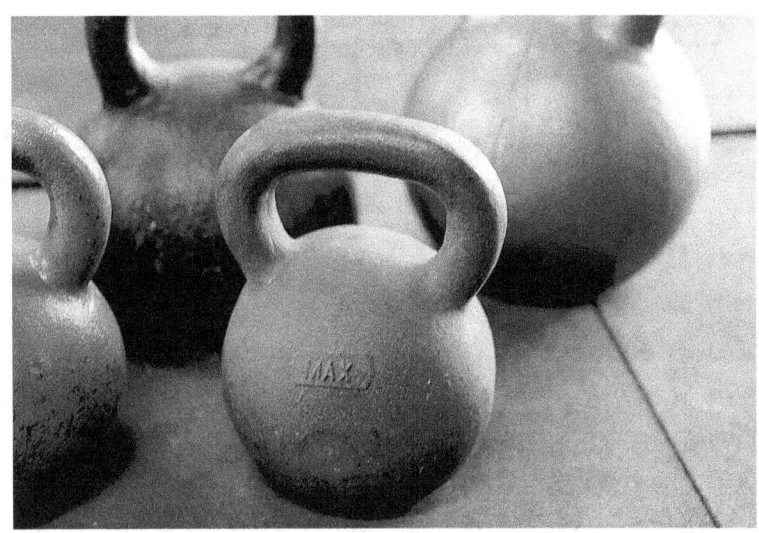

CHAPTER 1
Organizing Your Training Program

If you have read any of my early articles, you may be aware that I was extremely passionate about strength training as a kid growing up—so passionate, in fact, that I frequently overtrained. Focusing on program design in my college years, I created some overly complex programs. Using an old-fashioned, rigid model of periodization, I found it a crap shoot to hit new personal records at powerlifting meets or in the gym. Sometimes I would peak too early, sometimes I would peak too late, and sometimes I would, once again, overtrain.

There is no guaranteed route to success in strength training, but some programs are more efficient than others. The problem is that most people do not know where to begin. Of late, the trend in fitness and strength training has been to create lists of exercises, randomly thrown together, to form challenging workouts. Often, however, no thought is given to long-term planning or long-term training progress. These so-called "extreme workouts" do not always produce optimal outcomes. In order to create a program that will achieve your goals as safely and efficiently as possible, certain issues must be addressed. The first such issue is overload, which simply means pushing oneself to perform more work than before. Consistency and recovery also need to be examined. Simply put, it is almost always better to organize a workout according to a plan than to train in random fashion from a list of exercises.

While some programs are too random and others too rigid to allow for bumps along the way, there is a third option. To help us understand this third option, let's first briefly examine the program model I used early in my career which was very close to what is known as the Linear Model of Periodization, Linear Periodization, which is seldom used anymore in its pure form, divides training into different phases, or cycles, that focus on specific training outcomes. These programs typically include "macrocycles" of 9-12 months, "mesocylces" of 3-4 months, and "microcycles" of 1-4 weeks. Specific terminology may vary, but organization into an annual plan of cycles is the common factor. Though Linear Periodization provided the foundation for modern program design, as a program model it has several flaws. First, it does not allow for the simultaneous training of multiple attributes—such as strength, power, hypertrophy (muscle mass), or muscular endurance—that many sports require. In order to peak for one attribute, an athlete must sacrifice other attributes. Second, this model can very easily lead to overtraining since it can be quite rigid and training loads are determined well in advance, with little allowance for immeasurable variables such as stress, lack of sleep, illness and other factors. Last, peaking, which is the main purpose of the Linear Model, is very difficult to time effectively. Calculating a peak, the maximizing of performance at a specific point in time, is a true art form. Where many athletes may require multiple peaks throughout their sport season, strength enthusiasts usually require none at all. Why then should either athletes or strength enthusiasts train as though they need to be at their best at a single point in time when, in fact, it might be more practical to maintain a high degree of physical preparation almost year-round?

If the Linear Model of Periodization is the epitome of rigidity, the "complexes" and "high intensity intervals" that are in vogue these days are the other extreme, with almost no rhyme or reason. The purpose of training is to maximize the development of specific training attributes. We must ask ourselves if a given workout, even though it might be difficult, accomplishes this outcome. Many people, including professional coaches and trainers, think that if you vomit or are injured the workout must be a good one.

Regular training requires some form of organization. Good coaches do not simply pound their athletes into the ground. Simply put, training in extreme circuits does not take into account the specific relationship between the imposed stress and the recovery necessary to realize particular training outcomes. The best coaches have a plan. It may allow some degree of flexibility, but they will know what weaknesses need to be strengthened and have a strategy for addressing them.

An alternative model to Linear Periodization and random complexes is nonlinear, or undulating, periodization. Nonlinear periodization is a newer model of periodization that has emerged in part to address the needs of athletes who require multiple training attributes simultaneously for sports without defined peaks. Unlike the Linear Model, the Nonlinear Model of periodization is characterized by frequent alterations of training variables—such as intensity, density, and volume—with program alterations occurring monthly, weekly, or even daily. The purpose of these frequent adjustments is to more efficiently stimulate the neuromuscular system and improve recovery, thus maximizing training outcomes. The program, however, is absolutely not random. Exercise rotation, recovery, and adjustments are pre-planned to maximize training outcomes. Nonlinear periodization also allows for flexibility in timing sessions and assigning training loads. A realistic program needs to make room for unplanned circumstances like injury, illness, or a busy work schedule. Depending upon your specific program design, it may be possible to pick up where you left off if a workout is missed. Opponents of the nonlinear model maintain that mixed training produces mixed results. In the extreme, I would agree with this statement. Running marathons and powerlifting tend not to mix. However, my experience suggests that some attributes can be developed simultaneously and may even enhance one another.

Over the years, I have found that the best long-term progress comes from training maximal strength and power simultaneously. For the purpose of this book, let us define strength as the expression of the movement of an absolute load and power as the rate at which the work is completed. (Physicists and engineers, please bear with my overly simple definitions.) For example, assuming that movement speed and distance are the same, when two barbells are deadlifted, it can be said that the heavier barbell requires more strength. However, when maximal force is exerted, the movement of the faster barbell requires more power. In fact, a lighter weight, when lifted extremely fast, may require more power than the movement of a heavy weight. Though strength and power are related in practical terms, every seasoned lifter knows that possessing one does not guarantee great ability in the other. The bottom line is that a lifter can be strong, but slow and not very powerful. Conversely, a generally powerful person might lack great maximal strength. To maximize both attributes, however, one must be both powerful and strong. Therefore, both attributes must be trained.

The problem with training these attributes independently (a method called block training, in which one trains a single attribute exclusively for an average of three to six weeks) is that you will quickly begin to lose ability in other attributes. Block training in the short-term produces tremendous results, but if performed for more than a few weeks, injury or overtraining will likely occur. Block training also forces you to peak for a moment in time and leaves you ill prepared for unforeseen challenges that require attributes you are not currently training.

Personally, I have found a program with three or four primary training days, with the addition of extra "mini workouts" on off days, to be the most productive. If using three training days, a weekly training schedule might take the form of ABA or ABC. Session A would be dedicated to a specific attribute, session B dedicated to a different attribute, and session C might be a variation of A or B or something entirely different still.

If using a four-day program, I prefer a split routine with days 1 and 2 dedicated to power and days 3 and 4 dedicated to maximal strength. My personal routines have looked like this for some time; however, I have only recently added more variety in my heavy training. With this additional variety, I have realized even more progress with far less likelihood of overtraining.

With a simple programming framework, we still have an infinite number of ways to organize our specific workouts. In this book, I will outline a few of my favorite programs, with kettlebells as the primary tools, and fill in some gaps with other strength training tools such as dumbbells, bands, thick bars, traditional Olympic and power bars, hammers, stones, sandbags, and odd implements. Feel free to make changes as you see fit or as you feel necessary due to changes in your circumstances or goals. Keep in mind, however, that the spirit of this program is simultaneous training for both strength and power in order to maximize training outcomes, using kettlebells as the primary training implements.

For further reading:

Baker, D., Wilson, G., Carlyon, R. (1994). Periodization: The effect on strength of manipulating volume and intensity. *Journal of Strength and Conditioning Research* 8(4), 235-242.

Bounty, P., Campbell, B., Glavan, E., Cooke, ., and Antonio, J. (2011). Strength and conditioning considerations for mixed martial arts. *Strength and Conditioning Journal* 33(1), 57-67.

Buford, T., Rossi, S., Smith, D., and Wallace, A. (2007). A comparison of periodization models during nine weeks with equated volume and intensity for strength. *Journal of Strength and Conditioning Research* 21(4), 1245-1250.

Prestes, J., Frollini, A., de Lima, C., Donato, F., Foshini, D., Marqueti, R., Figueira, A., and Fleck, S. (2009). Comparison between linear and daily undulating periodized resistance training to increase strength. *Journal of Strength and Conditioning Research* 23(9), 2437-2442.

Rhea, M., Philips, W., Stone, W., Ball, S., Alvar, B., and Thomas, A. (2003). A comparison of linear and daily undulating periodized programs with equated volume and intensity for local muscular endurance. *Journal of Strength and Conditioning Research* 17(1), 82-87.

Simmons, Louie. (2007). *Book of Methods.* Westside Barbell.

CHAPTER 2
Introduction to the Main Lifts

The purpose of this section is to teach the basics of kettlebell training and build a foundation for the work in the following chapters. Do not take this section lightly. Many of the greatest kettlebell practitioners in the world use only these few basic lifts the majority of the time. Modern strength training legend John Brookfield was known to perform hundreds of heavy snatches throughout a workout. Nineteenth-century circus strongman Pyotr Kryloff was said to juggle 48-kilogram (106-pound) kettlebells among his many feats of strength. Unlike novice lifters, experts like these have virtually flawless technique. This allows them to train with both greater weight and greater overall volume than the beginner.

This early work will set the tone for your future kettlebell training. Remember: practice makes permanent. If you fail to develop proper technique in the beginning, it will be difficult to work on the advanced exercises that appear in later sections of this book. Conversely, the more you perfect your technique, the more efficient your movement patterns will become. This means that you will be able to lift heavier weights, perform more repetitions, and train harder and longer. So, even if you are in exceptional shape you should give this section one hundred percent of your attention and effort.

This section will give you examples of key kettlebell movements and assist you in making wise exercise selections and organizational choices. This is not to say that all foundational kettlebell exercises are included here. It is simply a beginning. For the more advanced kettlebell practitioner, this section offers a chance to examine exercises you may already know in greater detail, and to explore variations on fundamental techniques to which you might not have been previously exposed. Exercise order can be approached in multiple ways. Certainly large, whole-body exercises should be prominent in any kettlebell workout, though where in the workout they make their appearance may change depending upon circumstance or need. Assuming the exerciser is properly warmed up, large exercises that need to be emphasized should appear at, or near, the beginning of the workout.

UNIVERSAL ATHLETIC POSITION AND TWO-HANDED DEADLIFT

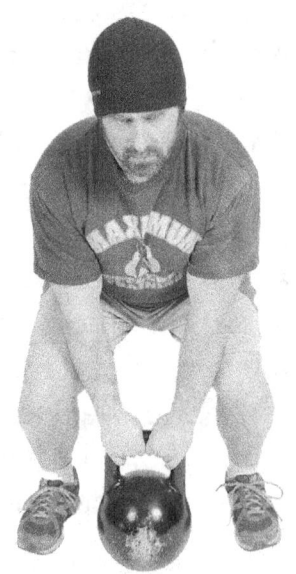

In athletics, the most common position of readiness is known as the Universal Athletic Position. It is the starting position that allows for the most efficient expression of movement and explosiveness. It consists of a flat back, where the spinal erectors that run along side the spinal column are contracted and the spine stable and protected. This does not mean that the back is perfectly upright, just that it is in a flattened position and not rounded. In addition the hips, knees, and ankles should be slightly flexed so that the shoulders are squarely over the knees. The core musculature of the midsection should be braced, or tightened, to protect the spine and aid in the transfer of momentum throughout the movement. This position is similar to that of a linebacker in American Football, ready to make a play. It is absolutely essential that you begin each lift in this Universal Athletic Position to avoid injury and master technique.

The Two-Handed Deadlift will teach you the posture of the Universal Athletic Position, which you will utilize for all of the major kettlebell movements and combinations. The Two-Handed Deadlift incorporates the large muscle groups of the thighs, hips, and lower back and can be performed with heavy weight, if available, as part of a workout or with lighter weight for a warm-up and or to practice basic posture and technique. Intermediate and advanced kettlebell practitioners may choose to skip the kettlebell deadlift during warm-up or may choose to periodically include heavier barbell deadlifts or stone-lifts as part of their regular programs.

Start by straddling the kettlebell and lining up your toes with the handle. Your feet should be slightly wider than your hips and pointed slightly outward. Keeping your feet flat, look straight ahead, then bend your knees and hips. This will allow you to keep your back in the proper alignment. As you drop your hips, keep your spinal erectors tight. This will aid in stabilizing your back and keeping you injury free. You will want a flat, relatively straight back. Grip the kettlebell with both hands, drive off of the floor, and stand up into a fully erect position, then lower the weight to the floor with control. Repeat this sequence of movements while maintaining a tight grip on the handle, until your set is completed. Continue to focus on your line of sight, posture, and braced core musculature throughout the set.

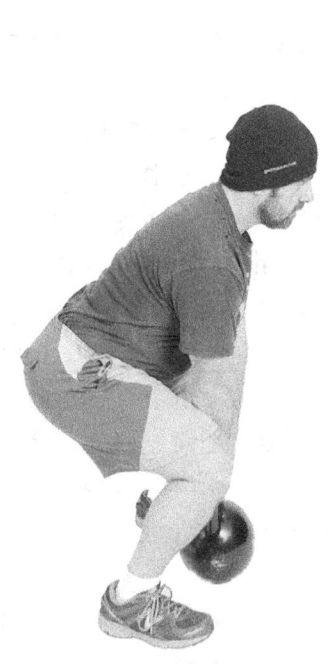
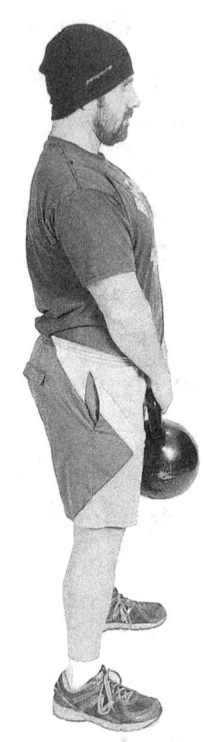

TWO-HANDED DEADLIFT: KEY POINTS

1. Straddle the kettlebell.
2. Toes lined up with the handle.
3. Feet slightly wider than hips and pointed out.
4. Eyes looking straight ahead.
5. Spinal erectors tight.
6. Bend knees then hips and drop into a squatting position.
7. Grip the kettlebell with both hands.
8. Keeping your arms straight, drive off of floor with hips, thighs, and lower back into erect position.

NOTE

Keep your line of sight neutral. Looking straight down may cause you to drop your head. This in turn will cause you to drop your shoulders and so on, until you are leaning forward, thus causing improper technique, excessive use of the low back muscles, and possibly low back strain. Remember to incorporate the large muscles of the thighs, which requires you to bend your knees as much as the movement allows. Another common mistake is raised heels and/or heel movement. If your heels are rising as you drop your hips to the floor, or if they are creeping inward with each repetition so that your feet end up turned out excessively, you may not be evenly distributing your body weight on your feet. You are likely placing too much weight on the front of your feet. A possible cause of uneven weight distribution may be an excessively horizontal upper back. Remember, you want a flat back for the deadlift, not one that is perpendicular to the floor as you squat. Another potential contributor to heel movement is over-tightness in the hip flexors, hip external rotators, and/or hamstrings. Muscular imbalance in these areas can create a misalignment in the skeleton causing improper mechanics and a disruption of proper technique. You may simply need to increase the flexibility of these muscle groups to improve technique.

NOTE: ONE-HANDED DEADLIFT

Like the Two-Handed Deadlift, the One-Handed Deadlift is a simple yet very valuable exercise. Though I do not often use this as a stand-alone exercise during a main training session, it is effective for getting the feel of a heavy kettlebell before attempting clean or snatch variations. It also works very well in combination with other, more advanced, kettlebell exercises. For example, the One-Handed Deadlift might begin a combination movement such as a One-Handed Deadlift, One-Handed High Pull, followed by a Clean. It might also be performed for several repetitions before attempting a limit (maximal effort) weight; for example, one or two repetitions of the One-Handed Deadlift, immediately followed by a limit Clean or Snatch. Except for the obvious exception of using one hand, per form this movement exactly as you would a Two-Handed Deadlift. Be sure to keep your hand and the kettlebell centered at all times.

TWO-HANDED HIGH PULL

The Two-Handed High Pull, also called the Squat Pull, is one of my all-time favorite exercises, kettlebell or otherwise. It is similar to the high pull performed by Olympic weightlifters as an assistance movement for cleaning or snatching a barbell. The High Pull is fairly easy to learn and utilizes most major muscle groups, including the thighs, hips, lower back, upper back, arm flexors, and shoulders. Because it forces you to create abdominal pressure in order to protect the spine and to allow for maximum transference of momentum, it also helps to develop a stable core. This is true of all major kettlebell lifts, but especially for the basic ballistic movements, of which this is the first. Ballistic refers to movements that are extremely explosive, abrupt, and powerful.

The High Pull is essentially the addition of an upright row to a deadlift. Set up as you would for the deadlift, with your toes in line with the handle, feet slightly wider than hips and toes pointed slightly outward. Create a neutral line of sight by looking at a fixed point in the distance. Your shoulders should be pulled back slightly and your upper back should be flat. Squat down and grip the kettlebell with both hands, then drive upward, extending your knees and your hips. Continue the movement by drawing your hands up your body toward your chin. This is the upright-row part of the movement. To keep your wrists from being injured, turn your elbows up and keep them higher than your hands. It will look like you are making a "V" at the top of the movement with your forearms. Then lower the kettlebell by fully extending your arms toward the floor and then bending your knees and hips. Just before the kettlebell reaches the floor, "bounce" it back up by ballistically changing direction. You will be using the muscles of the hips and thighs to accomplish this change of direction. As you rise up for the next repetition, you should feel the kettlebell almost float past your waist. Though this is a whole-body exercise, your legs should be doing most of the work to generate momentum.

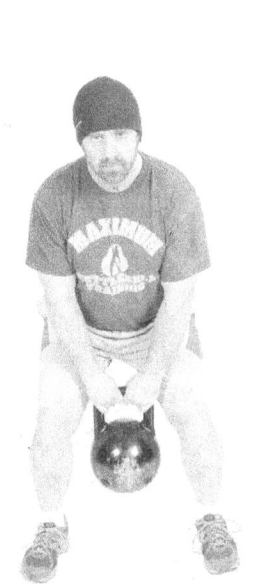
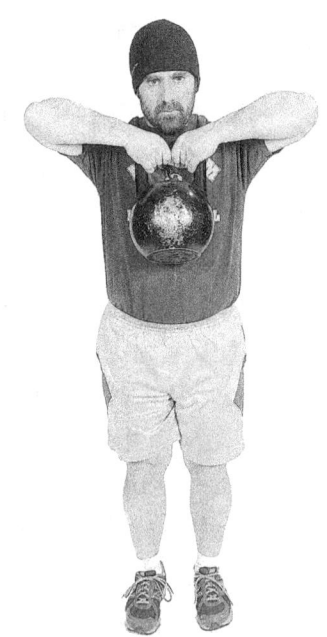

TWO-HANDED HIGH PULL: KEY POINTS

1. Set up same as you would for the deadlift.
2. Stand up to erect position, same as for the deadlift.
3. Continue movement by flexing elbows and drawing hands up ward toward chin.
4. Keep elbows turned up higher than hands.
5. Let arms fully extend on way down before bending knees and hips.
6. Just before hitting the floor, visualize hitting a spring and drive back up for the next repetition.

ONE-HANDED HIGH PULL

The One-handed High Pull variation is an excellent assistance exercise or preparatory exercise for the One-Handed Swing, One-Handed Clean, and the Single Snatch. Except for a few subtle differences, it is almost identical to the Two-Handed High Pull. Obviously you will be using one hand instead of two. You will also be forced to tilt slightly away from the kettlebell in order to center the weight between your knees. In addition, you will want to lean back and distribute a little of your bodyweight toward your heels as you lower the kettlebell between pulls. Using a heavy kettlebell, off center, with one hand tends to pull a lighter lifter forward so you will want to adjust your positioning as necessary to maintain your balance. Last, during the One-Handed High Pull the kettlebell may be pulled to chest height, as in the two-handed version, or to eye level. Pulling the weight to eye level is a particularly effective assistance exercise for heavy snatches.

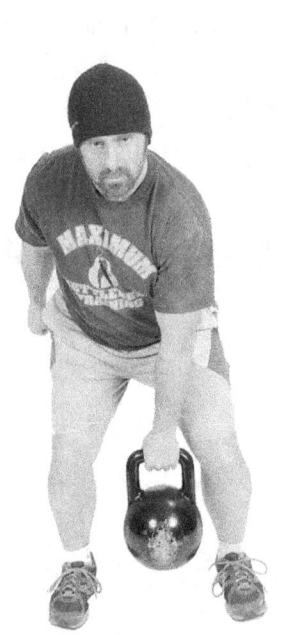
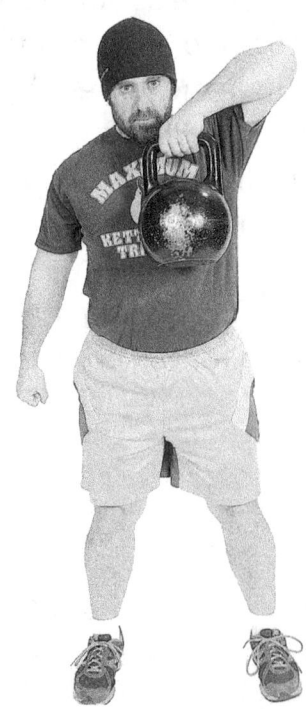

ONE-HANDED HIGH PULL: KEY POINTS

1. Set up same as you would for the One-Handed Deadlift.
2. Stand up to erect position, same as for the One-Handed Deadlift.
3. Continue movement by flexing elbow and drawing hand upward toward chin.
4. Keep elbow turned up higher than hands.
5. Let arms fully extend on the way down before bending knees and hips.
6. Just before hitting the floor, visualize hitting a spring and drive back up for the next repetition.

TWO-HANDED SWING: AMERICAN STYLE

The Two-Handed Swing is a great stand-alone exercise for beginning through advanced lifters. The Two-Handed Swing is an incredible exercise for developing explosiveness in the posterior chain musculature, great for inclusion in a speed program, where athletes focus on improving agility and quickness. In addition, the Two-Handed Swing is an excellent assistance exercise for deadlifts, squats, cleans, and snatches.

As with all the major power movements, line your feet with the kettlebell as you would for the deadlift. My preferred technique for this movement is to stand up as you would in a deadlift then lower your hips so that your hands are even with your knees. This is to help you get into the correct position and to avoid rounding your back. Next, swing the weight backwards through your knees to gain some momentum. This backswing will be referenced throughout this book. When the swing reaches its natural limit and your forearms are just beginning to brush against your thighs, forcefully extend your knees and hips. The momentum you generate by pushing off of the ground will be transferred into the weight, explosively moving the kettlebell forward and upward. Gently follow through with the arms and shoulders until the kettlebell is at eye level.

Your arms should be straight out from your body with the kettlebell lined up perfectly with your forearms. Let gravity pull the kettlebell toward the floor and swing it back between your legs. Bounce it back up for the next repetition by visualizing a spring behind you. This quick stretch, and then contraction of the muscles of the thighs, hips, and lower back will create a ballistic change in direction which, if performed properly, should feel very smooth.

Some years back, hardcore strength athletes gave the Kettlebell Swing a bad image, suggesting that it would ruin one's deadlift by causing a decrease in maximal strength since practitioners often used weights that were too light. This belief was incorrect. The fact is that the kettlebell has to be of appropriate weight to produce enough intensity to improve strength and power. For a super-heavyweight powerlifter, a 16-kiligram (35-pound) kettlebell swung for sets of 1,000 simply won't do the job. Choose your weights appropriately.

TWO-HANDED SWING: KEY POINTS

1. Straddle the weight with your feet slightly wider than hip width.
2. Line toes up with handle.
3. Get into squatting position with your back and feet flat.
4. Grip kettlebell with both hands.
5. Keep your head up and your line of sight neutral.
6. Stand up with the weight to get into position.
7. Slowly lower the kettlebell until your hands are even with your knees.
8. Swing backward to gain momentum.
9. Quickly extend your knees and hips, using the muscles of the thighs, hips, and lower back.

10. Follow through by raising your arms using the muscles of your shoulders until the kettlebell is at eye level. The kettlebell should be an extension of your body and lined up evenly with your arms. Let gravity pull the kettlebell down between your legs, with your hands passing through at knee level.

11. Ballistically change the direction of the movement at the mid-point, behind your hips, by using the muscles of the thighs, hips, and lower back and raise the kettlebell for next repetition.

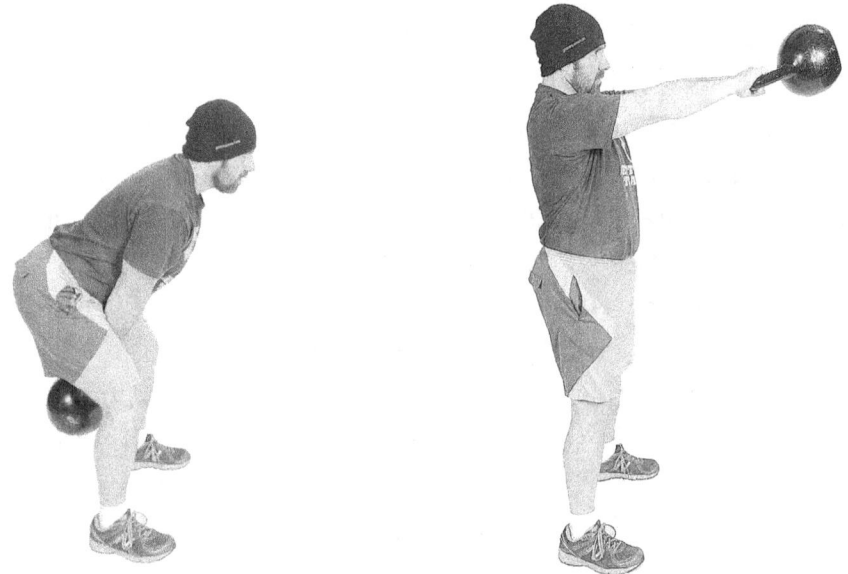

NOTE

Some trainers teach bringing the kettlebell past eye level to an over-head position. My opinion is that this increased range of motion does little to improve the benefit of the swing, since there is very little muscular force required for the lengthened part of the range. Lacking the punch and lockout technique of the Snatch, which I will introduce later, this style of swing increases the risk of over-flexion at the shoulder.

Note: Two-Handed Swing, Russian Style

The Russian-style Two-Handed Swing variation is similar to its American counterpart, except that it calls for significantly less knee flexion and extension. In this version, more emphasis is placed on hip and low back extension. This, in turn, places more emphasis on the hips and lower back musculature while decreasing the range of motion.

One-Handed Swing

Set-up for the One-Handed Swing is almost identical to that for the One-Handed High Pull, with the kettlebell centered between the knees. Grasping the kettlebell with one hand, begin with the same backswing as you would for the Two-Handed Swing, then drive the kettlebell forward and up in an arc, using the muscles of your lower back, hips, and thighs. Gently follow through with your shoulder until the kettlebell reaches eye level. Since you are using only one hand, your torso will be slightly tilted (as with the One-Handed High Pull) so that the kettlebell can pass between your knees. Be sure that you keep the kettlebell centered and lined up with the midline of your body throughout the movement to allow for maximum efficiency and safety. Using kettlebells that are heavy relative to your bodyweight may require you to adjust your center of mass and bodyweight distribution to maintain balance.

One-Handed Swing: Key Points

1. Set up as you would for the Two-Handed Swing.
2. Keep kettlebell centered.
3. Extend your knees and hips using the muscles of your thighs, hips, and lower back.
4. Follow through by raising your arm using the muscles of your shoulder until the kettlebell is at eye level.
5. Let gravity pull kettlebell down for next repetition.

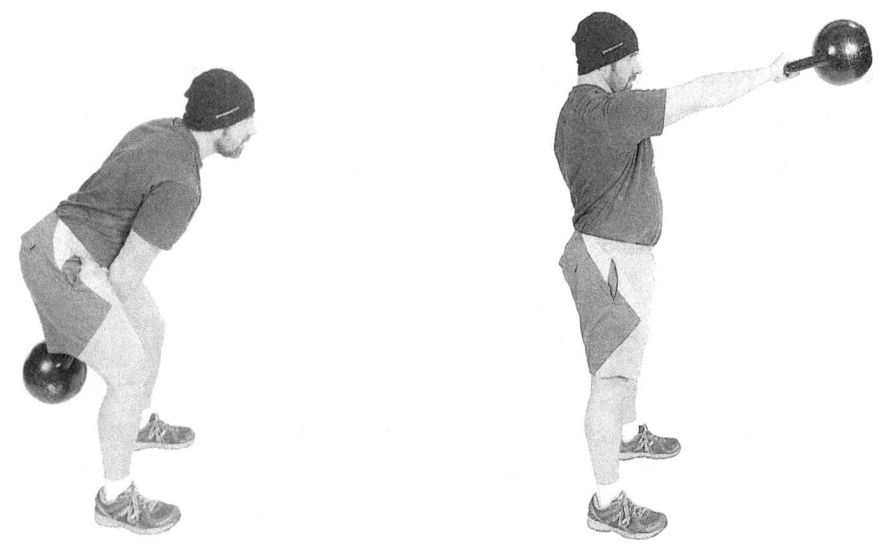

NOTE: ONE-HANDED SWING, RUSSIAN-STYLE

As with the Two-Handed Swing, the Russian-style One-Handed Swing calls for significantly less knee bend and extension than its American counterpart. In the Russian version more emphasis is placed on hip and lower back extension, with little emphasis on knee extension.

DOUBLE CLEAN

Of the several variations of the clean, I find the Double Clean the easiest to begin with. Simply put, a clean is a pull to a racked position outside of the shoulder. Double Cleans are usually easier to learn than single cleans because the upper body is upright and symmetrical. Therefore, you do not have to lean to the side as you would for a single clean.

First, line up two ketllebells so that the handles are in a straight line. Straddle the kettlebells and line your toes up with the handles. Your legs should be wide enough for the weights to clear but not so wide that you feel off balance. Keeping your head up and shoulders back, start your back swing. As you swing both kettlebells forward pull your elbows into your sides and begin to move your hands to the outside of your shoulders. This is the same movement you would use to open a coat. As you flip the kettlebells over your forearms, natural shelves will be created with your hands, elbows, and shoulders. Once the kettlebells are in the racked position, pause briefly, then tip your elbows up. This will allow you to re-align the kettlebells with your forearms and direct the kettlbells forward and downward. Allow the weights to swing between your knees, stretching the back, hips, and thighs, then bring them up for the next clean.

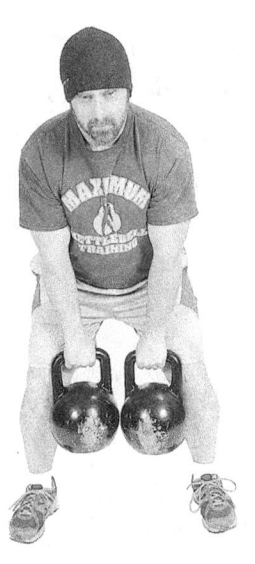
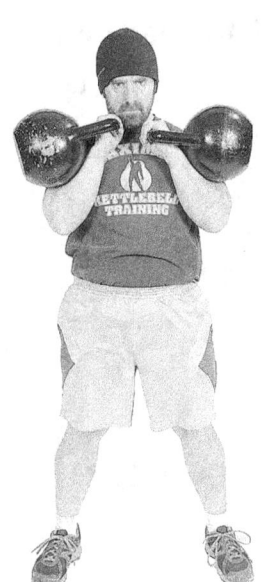

DOUBLE CLEAN: KEY POINTS

1. Line kettlebells up with handles in a straight line.
2. Straddle both kettlebells.
3. Start with backswing then bring kettlebells forward.
4. Pull elbows into your sides.

5. Move hands outward like you would to open a coat.
6. Flip kettlebells over onto the sides of your upper arms.
7. Pause briefly, then tip elbows up to direct kettlebells back between knees for next repetition.

DOUBLE SWING

The Double Swing, as its name indicates, is a swing using two kettlebells at once. This is a great exercise that will challenge your grip and coordination. The Double Swing is also a good exercise to perform when a single heavy kettlebell isn't available, or when you simply want to add variety to your routine.

Set up as you would for a Double Clean. Make your stance wide enough for the kettlebells to pass between your legs. An excessively wide stance, however, will throw you off balance. Keeping your head up and your shoulders back, start with a strong backswing to get the kettlebells moving. Extend your knees and hips and drive the kettlebells forward. Stand up to a fully erect position and follow through with the swing until the kettlebells reach eye level. Let gravity bring them down between your knees and allow the kettlebells to pass between your legs. Looking straight ahead will help keep you from being pulled forward. When the natural midpoint of the backswing is reached and you feel a slight stretch in your hips and lower back, extend your hips and knees, driving the kettlebells forward and up for the next repetition.

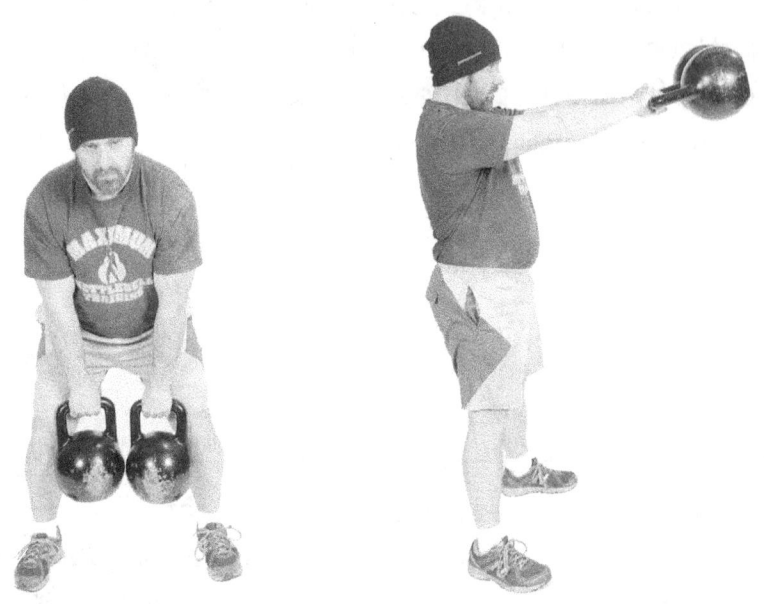

DOUBLE SWING: KEY POINTS

1. Set up as you would for a Double Clean.
2. Look straight ahead throughout the movement.
3. Utilize a strong backswing to start movement.
4. Extend knees and hips and swing.
5. When kettlebells reach eye level let gravity bring them down.
6. Allow kettlebells to pass knees, then spring back up for next repetition.

NOTE

It may be necessary to increase the width of your stance to accommodate two bells of moderate to large size.

ALTERNATING ONE-HANDED SWINGS

Alternating One-Handed Swings are an excellent variation of the One-Handed Swing and will challenge your grip strength, core development, and hand-eye coordination. Set up as you would for a traditional One-Handed Swing. Begin with the same backswing as you would for the One-Handed Swing, then drive the kettlebell forward and up in an arc, using the muscles of your lower back, hips and thighs. Gently follow through with your shoulder until the kettlebell reaches eye level. At this point, raise your free hand to the underside of the kettlebell handle with your palm facing upward. Then, cupping your hand and the kettlebell handle, slide your top hand off of the handle. You will now be gripping the kettlebell with your bottom hand. As you lower the kettlebell, rotate your hand so that your palm is now facing down. Let your arm fall as you would after a One-Handed Swing, then prepare for the handoff of the next repetition. Be sure to keep the kettlebell centered and lined up with the midline of your body throughout the movement.

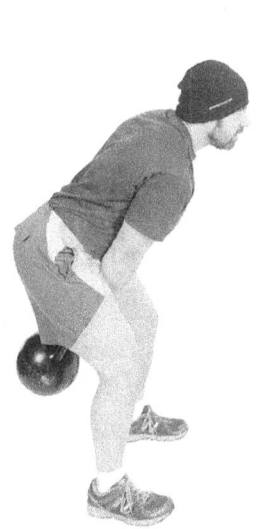
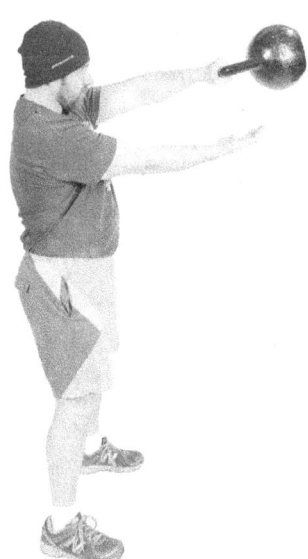

ALTERNATING ONE-HANDED SWINGS: KEY POINTS

1. Set up as you would for a One-Handed Swing.
2. Keep kettlebell centered.
3. Extend your knees and hips using the muscles of you thighs, hips, and lower back.
4. Follow through by raising your arm using the muscles of your shoulder until kettlebell is at eye level.
5. Switch hands by cupping the handle from the underside with your free hand.
6. Slide your top hand off of the kettlelbell handle.
7. Turn your new active hand palm down.
8. Let gravity pull kettlebell down for next repetition.
9. Alternate active hands.

ALTERNATING DOUBLE SWINGS

As with the Double Swing, you will use two kettlebells simultaneously for Alternating Double Swings. Challenging your core musculature and balance, the Alternating Double Swing is an effective assistance exercise for developing strength for Double Snatch and Double Clean variations.

Set up as you would for the Double Swing. Make your stance wide enough for the kettlebells to pass between your legs. Keeping your head up and your shoulders back, start with a strong backswing to begin the movement. Extend the knees and hips and drive one kettlebell forward. The other kettlebell will rise a bit, due to the extension of the knees, hips, and low back, but you will consciously raise only the kettlebell of the active arm. Stand up into a fully erect position and follow through with the swing until the kettlebell reaches eye level. Let gravity bring it down between your knees. Allow both kettlebells to pass between your legs. Looking straight ahead will help you from being pulled forward. When the natural midpoint of the rearward movement is reached and you feel a slight stretch in your hips and lower back, drive your hips forward and up then switch active sides for the next repetition. Alternate sides until your set is complete.

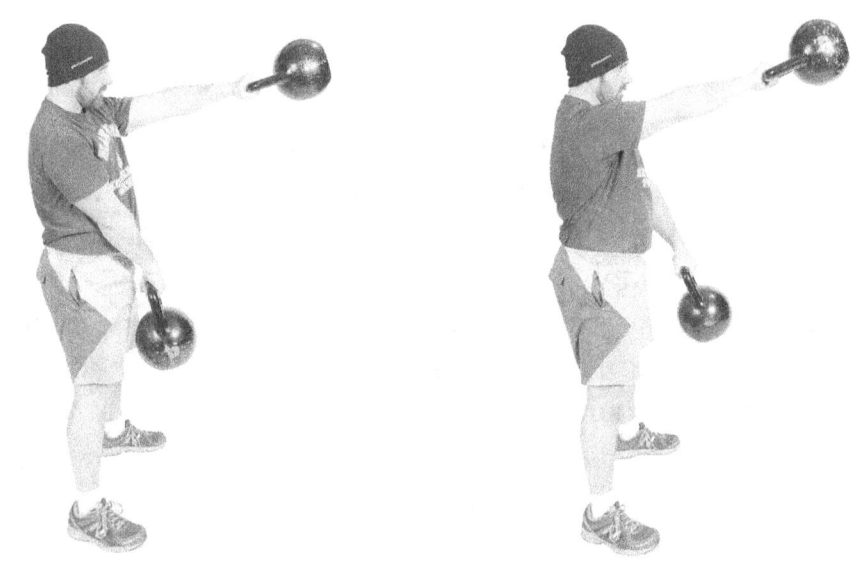

ALTERNATING DOUBLE SWINGS: KEY POINTS

1. Set up as you would for a Double Swing.
2. Look straight ahead throughout the movement.
3. Utilize a strong backswing to start movement.
4. Extend knees, hips, and low back and swing.
5. Raise only the active arm to eye level.
6. When kettlebell reaches eye level let gravity bring it down.
7. Allow both kettlebells to pass knees and switch active sides for next repetition.
8. Alternate active sides until set is complete.

NOTE

It may be necessary to increase the width of your stance slightly to accommodate two bells of moderate to large size.

CHAPTER 3
Cleans and Clean Variations: Beyond the Basics

Cleans are exercise variations that involve pulling a weight from the floor to a racked position on the shoulder or shoulders. In Olympic Weightlifting, a barbell is pulled from the floor to a resting position across the shoulders in front of the lifter's neck. Kettlebell cleans, however, more closely resemble kettlebell swings, where the lifter moves the weight in more of an arc-like pattern rather than the straighter line of movement of a Olympic barbell clean. In addition, all styles of kettlebell cleans require that the weights come to rest on the outside of the shoulders rather than on top of the shoulders.

Basic cleans are commonly performed in the Russian, or Girevoy, style or a MAX Kettlebell style. Russian style cleans are meant to be as mechanically efficient as possible to allow Russian kettlebell sport practitioners, known as Girevoy, to perform as many cleans as possible in competition. MAX kettlebell cleans, however, were developed to improve the high pull movement, from the knees to the chin, of athletes involved in grappling and other sports, where maximal power is required to draw an opponent toward the athlete's center mass, then explosively redirect their momentum.

SINGLE CLEAN: MAX VARIATION

The heavy Single Clean is probably my all-time favorite kettle-bell movement and is well worth learning because it translates beautifully to sports such as football, wrestling, judo ju jitsu, and many others. I initially developed this particular style of clean for grappling sports. It differs from a Russian-style clean in that it involves a larger range of motion and the kettlebell must rotate over your forearm instead of around it. Remember, a clean is a pull to a rack position on the outside of the upper arm and shoulder. Unlike a barbell clean, where the pull is almost completely vertical, the Single Clean begins like a Single Swing.

Start with a back swing, then, as the kettlebell moves forward, pull your elbow back into your side. Just as the kettlebell begins to flip over the back of your hand, lean to the side away from it. As the kettlebell rotates, give a quick shrug of your active shoulder to speed its movement. Move laterally instead of twisting back. It should almost look like you are ducking out of the way. This will push your hip out, helping to support the weight. As the kettlebell begins to make contact with your body, landing smoothly in the rack position, bend your knees slightly to absorb some of the shock. Do not allow your hand to go past your shoulder. Pause briefly, then tip your elbow up to re-align the kettlebell with your forearm and direct it forward and down for the next repetition.

SINGLE CLEAN MAX VARIATION: KEY POINTS

1. Set up as you would for a single swing.
2. Pull elbow to side as kettlebell reaches waist height.
3. Lean away from kettlebell as it flips over forearm.
4. Rack kettlebell on the outside of upper arm and shoulder.

5. Bend knees slightly to absorb shock as kettlebell comes into contact with body.
6. Tip elbow to direct weight toward floor for next repetition.

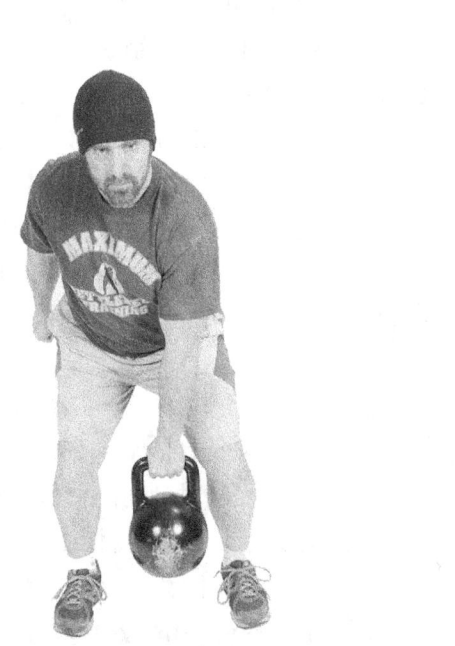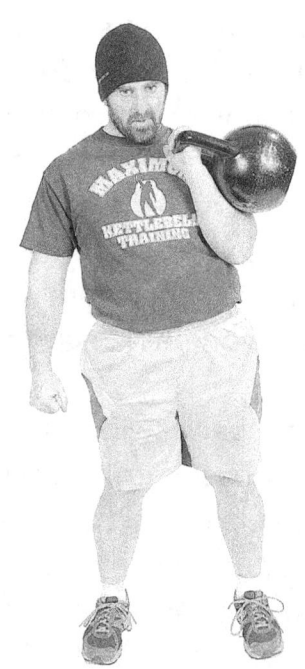

NOTE: RUSSIAN-STYLE CLEAN

The Russian-style clean variation is similar to its American counterpart but involves a shorter range of motion and a movement pattern that keeps the kettlebell closer to the body, thus less force is required to get the kettlebell in the rack position.

To perform the Russian-style clean, set up as you would for the American style, but instead of swinging wide, keep the kettlebell close to your body, then loop the kettlebell around your forearm, like you are throwing a coat over your shoulder. Your torso will remain in a more upright position using this technique. Like the Russian-style snatch, this technique was created to maximize mechanical efficiency for competition. Again, as with the swing and snatch techniques, try both and see what better suits your needs.

ALTERNATING CLEAN

The challenging Alternating Clean develops your grip, forearms, and cardiovascular system. The range of motion is short compared to other clean variations, which creates a need for explosiveness from the hips.

Set up as you would for the Double Clean. You can either stand up with both kettlebells or start with one already cleaned to a racked position. Regardless of how you start, at least one kettlebell needs to be lined up with the center of your body. I teach this exercise by telling my students to concentrate on cleaning the lower kettlebell. Gravity will help you lower the one on your shoulder. As you clean the bottom kettlebell, tip the elbow of the racked kettlebell up. This will re-align it with your forearm and help you move it forward and downward. When you drive up for the clean portion of this movement you will most likely extend your ankles as well as your hips and knees. This will bring you up on your toes, giving you some extra power to help compensate for the short range of motion. Try to get into a rhythm and just hop into each repetition.

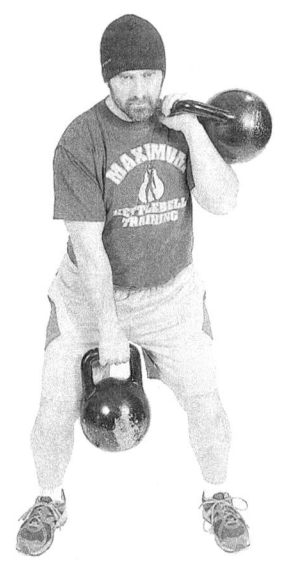
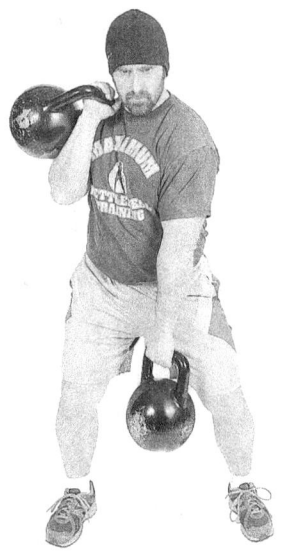

ALTERNATING CLEAN: KEY POINTS

1. Set up as you would for a Double Clean
2. Clean one kettlebell to racked position and center other between knees.
3. Bend knees and hips and clean the bottom weight. As it rises, tip your top elbow to lower the top kettlebell. These two movements should be simultaneous.
4. Performing Alternating Cleans resembles hopping in a rhythmical motion.

··

SINGLE OUTSIDE CLEAN

Though you will likely use less weight when performing the Single Outside Clean than you will for the MAX or Russian-style cleans, this is a great assistance exercise for developing maximal strength in any of the big power movements. The Single Outside Clean emphasizes speed and explosiveness in the upper part of the range of motion and in racking the kettlebell. Success in these parts of the movement is the difference between making and missing a heavy lift. Anyone who wants to advance in other styles of cleans should spend time on the Single Outside Clean. It is a great assistance movement.

Begin by standing with your feet hip-width, holding the kettlebell to the outside of your thigh. Looking straight ahead, bend both knees slightly until your hand is in line with your knees. At this point you will be leaning slightly to the weighted side. Extend your knees, hips, and low back and flex your elbow, quickly scooping the kettlebell into a racked position. Avoid leaning back excessively. Rather, concentrate on pulling the kettlebell straight up, then quickly shrugging and rotating your shoulder backward to rack the weight.

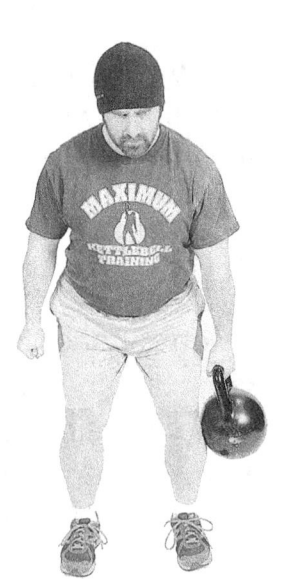 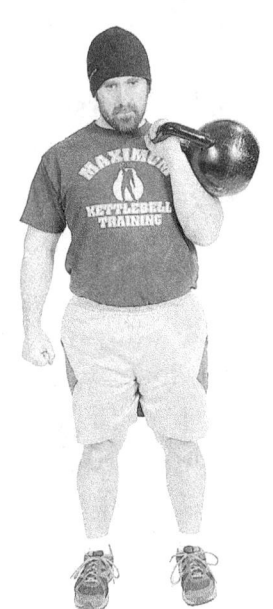

SINGLE OUTSIDE CLEAN: KEY POINTS

1. Set up with the kettlebell handle lined up with your toes on the outside of your foot. Your feet should be hip-width.
2. Grip the kettlebell, maintaining a flat back and neutral line of sight
3. Extend your knees and hips forcefully, and draw the kettlebell upward to chest height.
4. Quickly shrug your shoulder upward and backward in a circular motion, then pull the kettlebell into a racked position on the outside of upper arm and shoulder. This movement resembles a dumbbell cheater curl.
5. Bend knees slightly to absorb shock as kettlebell comes into contact with body.
6. Tip elbow to direct weight forward and downward for next repetition.

DOUBLE OUTSIDE CLEAN

The Double Outside Clean is very similar to the Single Outside Clean, except for the symmetry of handling two weights at once. Rather than leaning to either side, you will be forced to drive upward, evenly with both legs.

Begin by standing with your feet hip-width, holding the kettlebells to the outside of your thighs. Looking straight ahead, bend both knees slightly until your hands are in line with your knees. Then, extend your knees, hips, and low back and flex your elbows, quickly scooping the kettlebells into a racked position. Concentrate on pulling the kettlebells straight up, then quickly shrugging and rotating your shoulders backward to rack the weights.

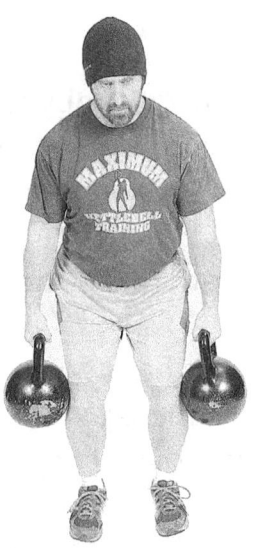
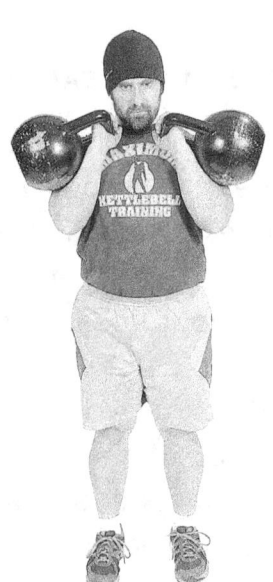

DOUBLE OUTSIDE CLEAN: KEY POINTS

1. Set up with the kettlebell handles lined up with your toes on the outside of your feet and your feet hip-width.
2. Grip the kettlebells, maintaining a flat back and neutral line of sight.

3. Extend your knees and hips forcefully, drawing the kettlebells upward to chest height.
4. Quickly shrug your shoulders upward and backward in a circular motion, then pull the kettlebells into a racked position on the outside of upper arms and shoulders. This movement resembles a dumbbell cheater curl.
5. Bend knees slightly to absorb shock as kettlebells come into contact with body.
6. Tip elbows to direct weights forward and downward for next repetition.

NOTE: DOUBLE CLEAN JUMPS

Adding a jump to the Double Clean further increases the difficulty of the exercise but also aids in the development of power in the hips and thighs. First, line up two ketllebells so that the handles are in a straight line. Straddle the kettlebells and line up your toes with the handles. Your legs should be wide enough to clear the weights but not so wide that you feel off balance. Keeping your head up and shoulders back, start your back swing. As you swing both kettlebells forward pull your elbows into your sides and begin to move your hands to the outside of your shoulders. This is the same movement you would use to open a coat. As you flip the kettlebells over your hands, your forearms, elbows, and shoulders will create natural shelves. The moment the kettlebells are in the racked position, immediately jump straight up as high as you can. When you land back on your feet, bend your knees and hips slightly to absorb some of the shock, then after pausing briefly, tip your elbows up, which will allow you to realign the kettlbells with your forearms in preparation for the next repetition. Allow the weights to swing between your knees, stretching your back, hips, and thighs, then bring them up for the next clean and jump.

CHAPTER 4
Snatch: The Undisputed King of Kettlebell Lifts

SINGLE SNATCH

The Single Snatch is considered by many practitioners to be the king of all kettlebell movements. Its huge range of motion goes from the floor to arm's length overhead. It uses almost all of the major muscle groups, and it demands an explosive execution that translates well to many sports. Because of these traits, the Single Snatch perfectly blends strength and power while raising the heart-rate to near maximum levels.

If you have been practicing the High Pull and Swing variations you should be well prepared to work on Snatches. Again, set up with the Universal Athletic Position, with your feet slighlty wider than hip-width, back flat, and bent knees and hips. Grip the weight with one hand so that it hangs just below knee level.

Begin the Snatch by taking a large backswing to get the kettlebell moving. Unlike the Swing, however, the Snatch has to come over-head for a full lockout, so you must generate significantly more power to accommodate the larger range of motion. This explosion must begin at the very bottom of the movement if you are to suc-cessfully complete the Snatch. You will need to continue to drive with your whole body throughout the entire range of motion.

To rack, or catch, the kettlebell overhead, you must make the weight roll gently onto your forearm by pushing into the handle approximately 12 inches before you reach the top of the movement, where your elbow will be fully extended. This pushing motion will turn the handle under the kettlebell, making for a soft landing in the racked position.

Once the kettlebell is locked out straight overhead, tip your wrist forward, so the kettlebell is once again aligned with your forearm. In this position, you have complete control of the weight and you can direct it freely. If you would simply lower your arm from the overhead position, without tipping the kettlebell forward, it would flop off of your forearm around shoulder height and jerk your body forward, pulling you off balance.

Snatches and other overhead lifts may sound complicated (or possibly borderline insane) but they are not as difficult in practice as they may sound in a written description, and they are well worth the brief learning curve. When snatches are executed correctly they are smooth, fluid, and have almost no impact on the forearm. Getting the feel of the movement takes a little practice. Trust your instincts. When snatches begin to feel easier and more fluid, you are likely on your way to perfecting your technique.

SINGLE SNATCH: KEY POINTS

1. Set up same as you would for single swing.
2. Use forceful backswing to gain momentum.
3. Extend the knees and hips using the muscles of the knees, hips, and low back.
4. Be explosive throughout entire movement.
5. Follow through and extend your arm overhead by using the muscles of the shoulder to drive past eye level.

6. Push into kettlebell just before top of movement so that ball rotates under handle and kettlebell gently rolls onto forearm.

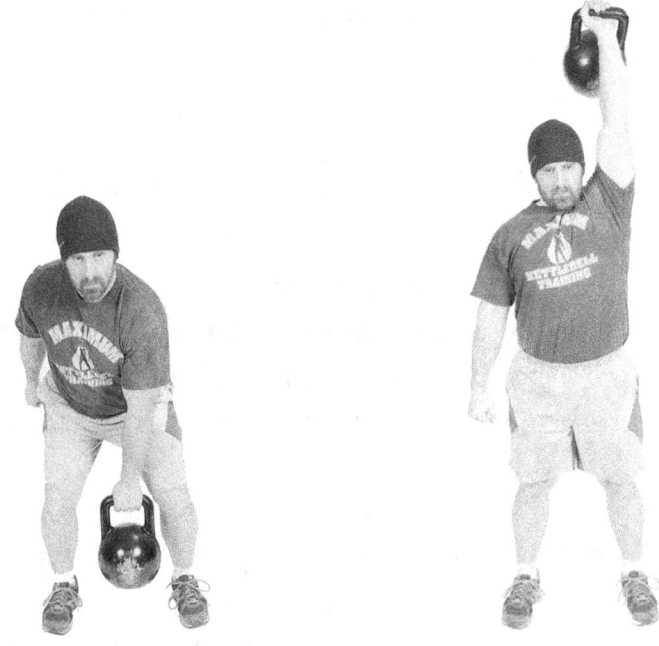

NOTE

The Russian-style Snatch variation is similar to its American counterpart but involves a shorter range of motion and a narrower swing that keeps the kettlebell closer to the body, thus less force is required to get the kettlebell in the racked position. To perform the Russian-style Snatch, set up as you would for the American-style, but instead of swinging wide, keep the kettlebell closer to your body and stand up just a bit straighter than you would in the American-style. Then, loop the kettlebell around your forearm into the racked position. This version of the Snatch was created for the sake of mechanical efficiency, so kettlebell sport athletes could maximize their repetitions when competing. Again, as with the Swing and Clean variations, try different styles and see what better suits your needs.

DOUBLE SNATCH

The Double Snatch is performed with two kettlebells. Set up as you would for a Double Clean. Keeping your head up and your shoulders back, take a forceful back swing. Explode forcefully from the back swing and drive with your whole body. When the kettlebells are approximately 12 inches from the overhead position, push into the handles as you would for a single snatch. If executed properly, there should be very little impact on the forearms. At this point, lower the kettlebells to your shoulders then tip your elbows to realign the kettlebells with your forearms, as you would for a Double Clean. Lowering the kettlebells to your shoulders before finishing the swing will keep you from being thrown off balance by the added weight. Move your arms forward and downward, then swing the kettlebells between your knees and explode back up for the next repetition.

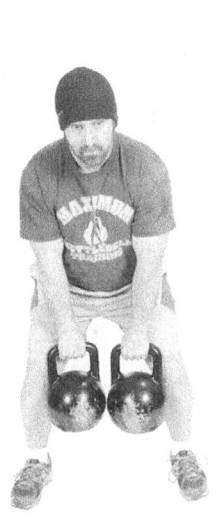
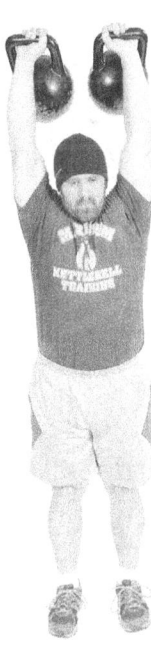

DOUBLE SNATCH: KEY POINTS

1. Set up as you would for the Double Clean.
2. Use strong backswing.
3. Snatch both kettlebells as you would for Single Snatch.
4. Push into kettlebells 12 inches before top of movement.
5. Lower kettlebells to shoulders before tipping down into next repetition.

....

ALTERNATING SNATCHES

As with the Alternating Clean, you will be using two kettlebells at once for Alternating Snatches. Heavy Alternating Snatches are arguably one of the toughest kettlebell exercises of them all. They are excellent for developing whole-body strength and they require absolute concentration.

Set up as you would for the Alternating Clean, with your feet slightly wider than your hips and your hands approximately knee height. With a strong, although short, backswing, snatch one kettlebell. Then tip the wrist of your active side forward to realign it with your forearm and begin to lower the top kettlebell. As the top kettlebell moves forward, explosively extend your ankles, knees, and hips and snatch the second kettlebell. Like Alternating Cleans, Alternating Snatches resemble a hopping motion. Concentrate on snatching the lower kettlebell. Gravity will help you lower the one overhead. Continue alternating sides until your set is complete.

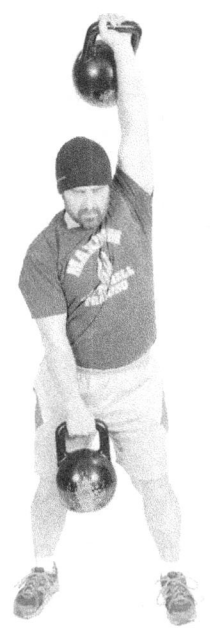
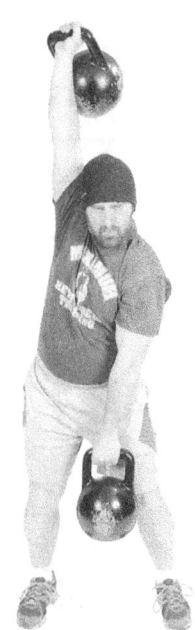

ALTERNATING SNATCHES: KEY POINTS

1. Set up as you would for an Alternating Clean.
2. Snatch one kettlebell to racked position overhead and center other between knees.
3. Tip your top wrist forward to realign the top kettlebell with your forearm and begin to lower the kettlebell.
4. As the top kettlebell moves foreward, extend your ankles, knees, and hips and snatch the bottom weight. These two movements should be simultaneous.
5. Like Alternating Cleans, Alternating Snatches resemble a rhythmical hopping motion.

CHAPTER 5
Overhead Press, Push Press, and Jerk Variations

TWO-HANDED OVERHEAD PRESS

There are many variations of the overhead press. The Two-Handed Overhead Press is a good one to begin with because it requires a little less balance than some of the others. Success with this exercise will build up your confidence for more advanced presses. Don't let the simplicity of this movement fool you, however. It can be extremely challenging once you reach near-limit weight. Like some of the stone pressing featured in strongman contests, the Two-Handed Kettlebell Press forces the lifter to not only press upward with the triceps and shoulders, but also inward with the forearms and the chest.

Begin by tipping the kettlebell on its side with the handle facing away from your body. Grip it around the ball with your thumbs wrapped tightly around the handle. As you pick it up, tip it back over so that the handle is now resting on the top of your chest. Your hands should be underneath the kettlebell, with the handle parallel to the ground and your elbows tucked into your sides. Bend your knees slightly to keep excessive strain off of your lower back. Keeping your line of sight neutral, press the kettlebell straight over your head. Pause briefly at the top then slowly lower the kettlebell down to your chest.

All Overhead Press variations can be performed with a pause in the bottom position to emphasize the starting strength required to perform the movement. Simply hold the kettlebell(s) in the bottom position for a 1–3 second pause before beginning the press. (If your aim is to build stamina, however, you should continue without pausing).

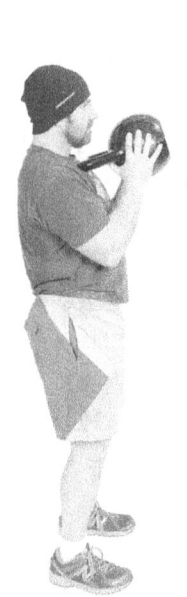 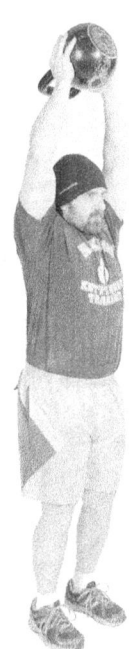

TWO-HANDED OVERHEAD PRESS: KEY POINTS

1. Hold kettlebell by its sides so that the handle is resting on your chest and your thumbs are wrapped around it.
2. Bend knees slightly.
3. Keep line of sight neutral and press kettlebell straight overhead.
4. Pause briefly then slowly lower to chest.

SINGLE OVERHEAD PRESS

The next pressing exercise you will add to your arsenal is the Single Overhead Press. Clean the kettlebell to a racked position on the outside of your upper arm. Take a hip width, or slightly wider, stance and turn your head so that you are able to look at the weight. This will help you keep your balance. The elbow of your active arm should begin in a low position and be tucked into your side. You may choose to brace your inactive hand against your hip or hold your arm straight out. Lean slightly away from the kettlebell, so that your hip helps to support the weight. Press to full overhead extension. If your body is properly aligned, an observer would be able to draw an imaginary line from the kettlebell to the center of your stance. Pause briefly, then slowly lower the weight until your elbow is once again tucked into your side. Once the kettlebell is resting in the racked position, pause if appropriate, then begin your next repetition.

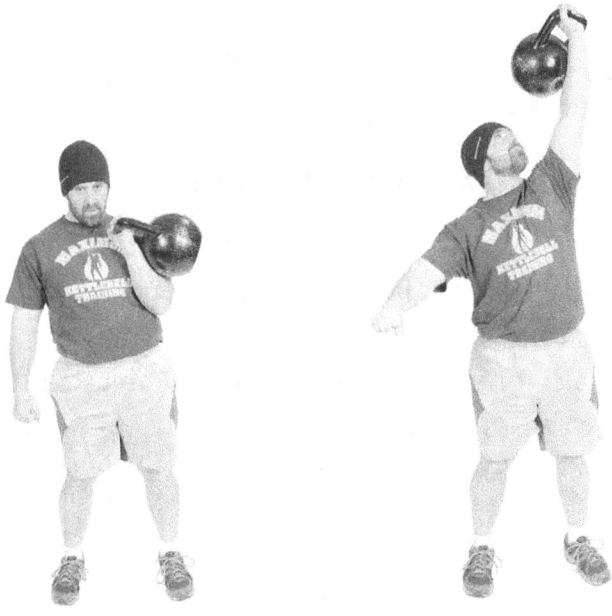

SINGLE OVERHEAD PRESS: KEY POINTS

1. Clean the kettlebell to a racked position (resting on the outside of your upper arm, with your elbow tucked into your side.)
2. Stance should be slightly wider than shoulder width.
3. Turn head and look at kettlebell for balance.
4. Follow kettlebell with your eyes to help maintain balance.
5. Press to full overhead extension, with the kettlebell directly over the center of your stance.
6. Pause briefly.
7. Slowly lower kettlebell until elbow is tucked into your side.

....

DOUBLE OVERHEAD PRESS

Clean the kettlebells to the outside of your shoulders as you would for a Double Clean. Bend your knees slightly and tighten your stomach to stabilize your lower back. Your elbows should be tucked into your sides. Looking straight ahead, take a deep breath then exhale and press the kettlebells to a full overhead extension. Pause briefly, then lower the kettlebells until they are once again on the sides of your shoulders. Your elbows should, once again, be tucked into your sides. After a brief pause, continue pressing the kettlebells until your set is compete.

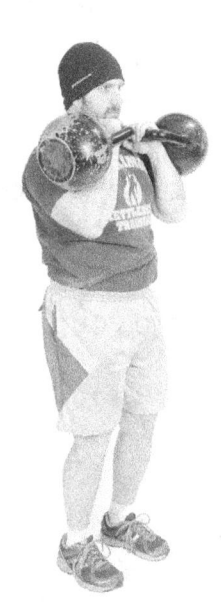 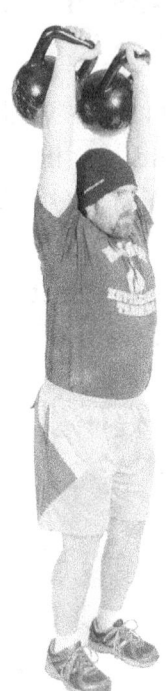

DOUBLE OVERHEAD PRESS: KEY POINTS

1. Clean kettlebells to sides of shoulders.
2. Look straight head, tighten abdominal muscles, and slightly bend knees.
3. Take deep breath, then press while exhaling.
4. Fully extend your arms.
5. Pause briefly at top then slowly lower weights until kettlebells are into starting position.
6. Pausing once again in the starting position, then continue pressing the kettlebells overhead until your set is complete.

ALTERNATING OVERHEAD PRESS

Clean the kettlebells to the outside of your shoulders as you would for a Double Clean. Slightly bend your knees and tighten your abdominal muscles to stabilize your spine. Take a deep breath then press one kettlebell overhead. Pause briefly, then lower the first kettlebell to the starting position. As you lower the first kettlebell, begin to press the second kettlebell overhead. Continue to alternate sides until your set is complete.

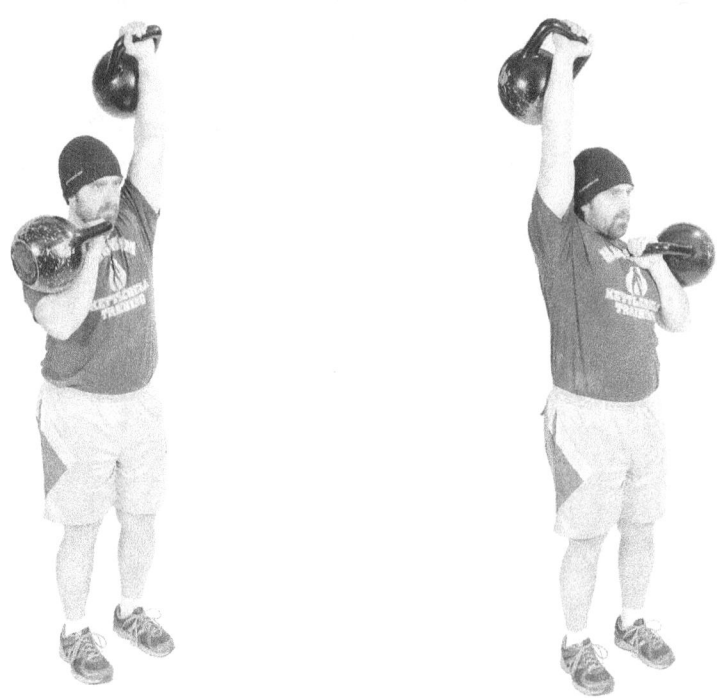

ALTERNATING OVERHEAD PRESS: KEY POINTS

1. Set up as you would for the Double Overhead Press.
2. Slightly bend knees and tighten abdomen.
3. Press one kettlebell to full overhead extension.
4. As you lower the first kettlebell, begin pressing the second.
5. Continue to alternate until set is complete.

ONE-STAYS-UP OVERHEAD PRESS

In this variation of the press, one kettlebell will be fully extended overhead at all times. This exercise effectively works the small stabilizing muscles of the rotator cuff, triceps, and shoulders. Fatigue tends to set in quickly.

Clean the kettlebells to the outside of your shoulders as you would for a Double Clean. Slightly bend your knees and tighten your abdominal muscles to stabilize your spine. Take a deep breath then press both kettlebells overhead. Keeping one arm extended, bring the other kettlebell down until your elbow is tucked into your side. Press it back up and pause briefly with both kettlebells fully extended overhead. Continue to alternate sides until your set is complete.

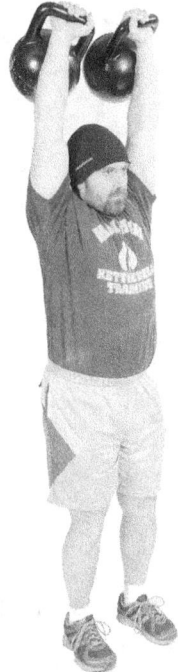 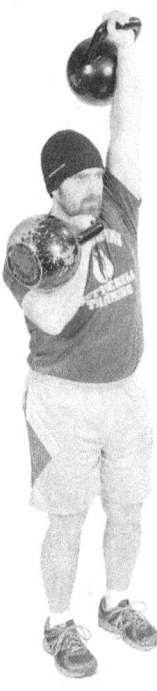

ONE-STAYS-UP OVERHEAD PRESS: KEY POINTS

1. Set up as you would for the Double Overhead Press.
2. Slightly bend knees and tighten abdomen.
3. Press both kettlebells to full extension.
4. Keeping one arm extended, lower the other kettlebell.
5. Press kettlebell back up, pause; then lower the other kettlebell.
6. Continue to alternate until set is complete.

SINGLE AND DOUBLE BOTTOMS-UP PRESS

This exercise is awesome for developing crushing grip strength as well as stability in the muscles of your trunk. You can grip the kettlebell anywhere on the handle you wish as long as the kettlebell is upside down.

Set up as you would for a Single or Double Press, with one or two kettlebells. Grip the handle(s) as tightly as you can and clean the kettlebell(s) into the rack position. Slowly press the kettlebell(s) to full extension and very slowly lower it back to your shoulder. Continue pressing in this fashion until you have completed your set, then lower kettlebell(s) to the floor.

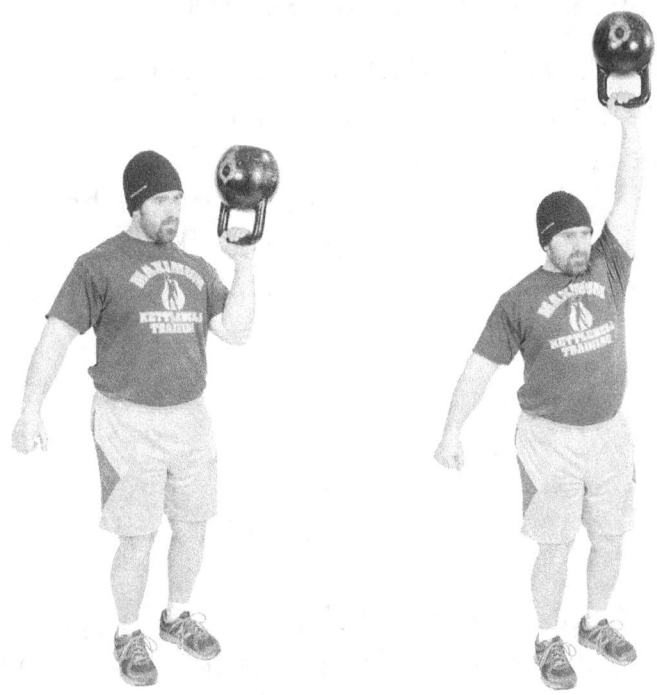

SINGLE AND DOUBLE BOTTOMS-UP PRESS: KEY POINTS

1. Use a moderate weight.
2. Set up as you would for a single or double press, with one or two kettlebells.
3. Grip handle(s) as tightly as possible.
4. Clean kettlebell(s) to a rack position with the kettlebell upside down.
5. Maintaining balance, slowly press kettlebell(s) to full extension.
6. Slowly lower kettlebell(s) to shoulder and repeat series of movements until set is finished.

NOTE: PUSH PRESS AND JERK VARIATIONS

Push-press and Jerk variations are a way to use slightly heavier weights for your pressing exercises. Both require using your legs to provide additional help in lifting the kettlebell.

To perform a Push-Press, take a hip-width or slightly wider stance. Bend your knees then quickly straighten them to gain momentum and drive the kettlebell into a full extension, overhead. The addition of the knee bend and extension in this technique allows you to use more weight than you would for a basic press.

To perform a Jerk, begin as you would for a Push-Press by taking a hip-width or slightly wider stance. Bend your knees then quickly straighten them to gain momentum. As the weight leaves your shoulder, continue pressing up, while simultaneously bending your knees and hips, so that you duck under the weight. Your goal is to both push and drop at the same time. Once the kettlebell is in full overhead extension, extend your knees and hips, rising to a fully erect position. Lower kettlebell to your shoulder to prepare for the next repetition. The addition of the simultaneous leg drive, arm extension, and bodydrop in this technique allows the experienced lifter to press with more weight than either the basic presses or the Push-Pull allow for.

CHAPTER 6
Bentover Row Variations

BENT-OVER ROW

The Bent-Over Row is the first major movement dedicated to the upper back. As the name implies, this is a pull, or row, in the bent-over position. It can be performed with a variety of grips and stances, depending on what part of your upper back and shoulders you wish to emphasize. To begin, however, I recommend the following standard foot and hand positioning. With the kettlebell on the floor, step back so that it is even with your front foot. The handle should be parallel with the side of your foot and your feet should be pointing in the same direction. Brace yourself by placing the hand of your forward side on your thigh. Bend at your waist so that your upper body is almost parallel to the ground. Grip the kettlebell with your free hand and pull the handle to your ribs without twisting your upper body. Lower the kettlebell almost to the floor and repeat for the next repetition. When you are finished with your set on one side, reverse your position and repeat on the other.

BENT OVER ROW: KEY POINTS

1. Stagger your step approximately a stride length so that your feet are straight ahead and parallel.
2. Bend at your waist and brace yourself by placing your forward hand on your thigh.
3. Grip the kettlebell with your free hand and pull to your ribs with-

out twisting your upper body.

4. Lower almost to floor and repeat.

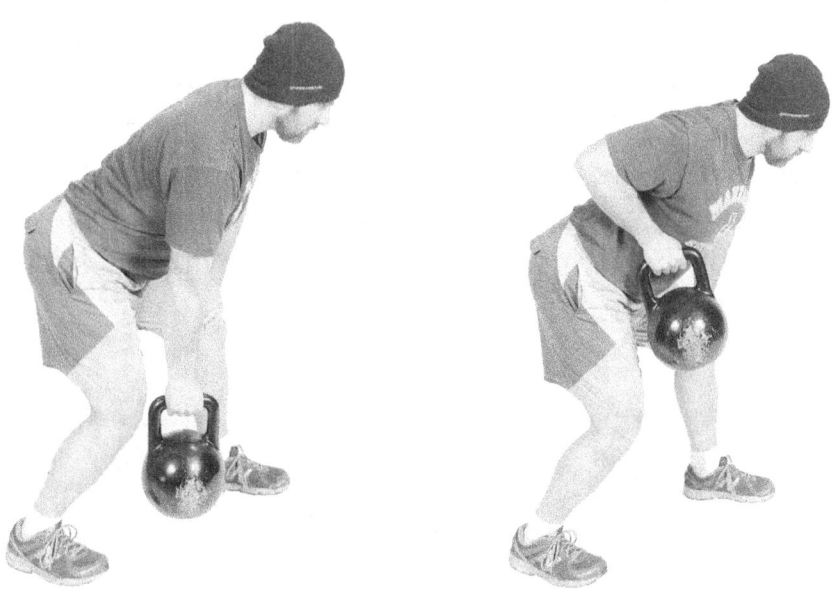

NOTE

A common positioning error is to turn the back foot outward. This usually causes rotation of the hips, which in turn leads to rotation of the shoulders. To avoid this, double-check to ensure that your back foot is pointed straight ahead.

Several grip variations can be used for the Bent-over Row and other row variations, depending upon what muscles you would like to emphasize. All variations will work the upper back; however, you can also target your biceps, rear shoulder, or the outside of the large upper back musculature. For the biceps you can use a supine (palms up) grip. For the rear shoulder you can use a prone (palm down) grip with your elbows flared out. Lastly, to emphasize the large lattisimus (upper back) muscles you can use a neutral (palms in) grip and keep your elbows tight to your sides.

DOUBLE ROW

The Double Row is another simple, yet very effective, kettlebell exercise for the upper back. Set up as you would for a Double Clean by gripping both kettlebells. Stand up to a fully erect position, then bend at your waist and knees until your upper back is slightly lower than a 45-degree angle. Tighten your abdomen and spinal erectors so that your spine is stable. While looking straight ahead, draw the weights up to your ribs and pause briefly. Slowly lower the kettlebells until your arms are fully extended, with the kettlebells inside of your knees.

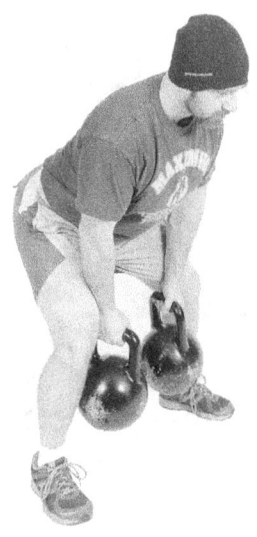 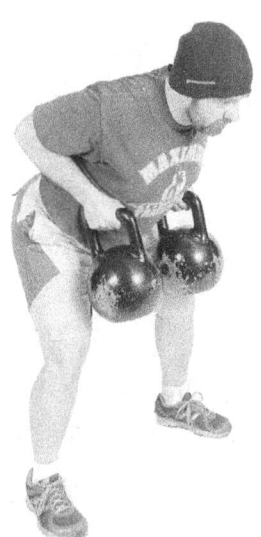

DOUBLE ROW: KEY POINTS

1. Set up as you would for a Double Clean.
2. Grip weights and stand up to a fully erect position.
3. Slowly bend at the waist and knees until your upper body is slightly lower than a 45-degree angle to the floor.
4. Tighten muscles of your trunk.
5. Pull your hands to your ribs and pause briefly.
6. Slowly lower the kettlebells until your arms are fully extended.

ALTERNATING (SEE-SAW) ROW

The Alternating Row is yet another very effective kettlebell exercise for the upper back. Set up as you would for a Double Row by gripping both kettlebells. Stand up to a fully erect position, then bend at your waist and knees until your upper back is slightly lower than a 45-degree angle. Tighten your abdomen and spinal erectors so that your spine is stable. While looking straight ahead, draw one kettlebell to your ribs. As you lower the that kettlebell toward the floor, begin to draw the second kettlebell to your ribs. Repeat alternating rows until your set is complete.

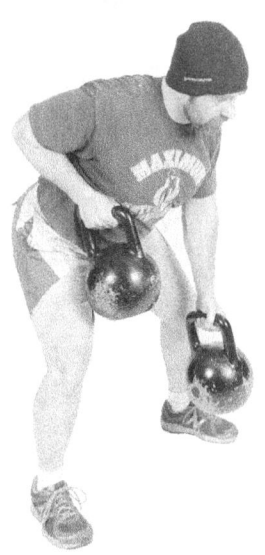 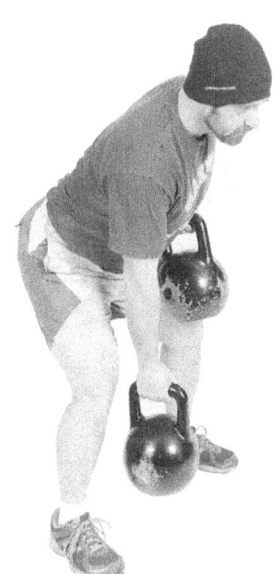

ALTERNATING (SEE-SAW) ROW: KEY POINTS

1. Set up as you would for a Double Row.
2. Grip weights and stand up to a fully erect position.
3. Slowly bend at the waist and knees until your upper body is slightly lower than a 45-degree angle to the floor.
4. Tighten muscles of your trunk.
5. Lift one kettlebell to your ribs.
6. As you lower the first kettlebell, begin to lift second kettlebell to your ribs.
7. Repeat alternating motion until set is complete.

ONE-STAYS-UP ROW

Like the other row variations, the One-Stays-Up Row emphasizes the upper back muscles. Line up two kettlebells as you would for a Double Row. Pull up both kettlebells to your ribs then, keeping your shoulders level, lower one kettlebell until your arm is completely extended. Pull that kettlebell back to your ribs, pause briefly, then lower the second kettlebell to a fully extended position. Continue to alternate the kettlebells in this fashion until your set is complete.

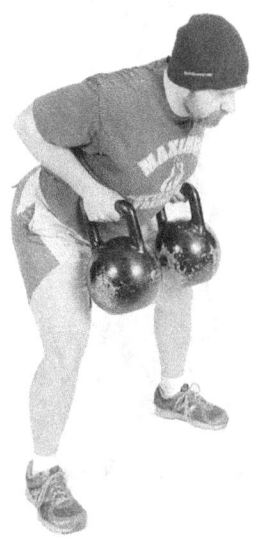
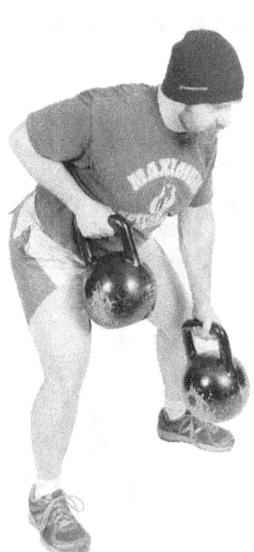

ONE-STAYS-UP ROW: KEY POINTS

1. Line up two kettlebells just inside your feet as you would for a Double Row.
2. Bend at your waist and knees as you normally would for a Double Row.
3. Pull both kettlebells to your midsection.
4. Lower one kettlebell until your arm is fully extended.
5. Pull it back up to your midsection.
6. Pause briefly then lower the opposite kettlebell.
7. Continue to alternate rowing kettlebells until your set is complete.

CHAPTER 7
Floor Press Variations

TWO-HANDED FLOOR PRESS

The first of the floor press series, the Two-Handed Floor Press is a simple yet effective exercise that works the muscles of the chest, shoulders, and triceps. The round shape of the kettlebell adds an extra challenge because you must push in as well as up when pressing. The Two-Handed Press is typically considered a beginner's exercise. When you outgrow it, simply move on to the Single Floor Press or another variation. To begin, lie flat on your back and pull the kettlebell onto your chest so that it is on its side with the handle toward your chin. Grip the kettlebell on its sides with your thumbs wrapped around the handle. Press the kettlebell straight over your chest to arm's length. Slowly lower the kettlebell then repeat until your set is completed.

TWO-HANDED FLOOR PRESS: KEY POINTS

1. Lie flat on your back.
2. Pull a kettlebell onto the center of your chest with the handle pointed toward your chin.
3. Hold with thumbs wrapped around the handle.
4. Press to arm's length.
5. Pause briefly at the top position then slowly lower and repeat.

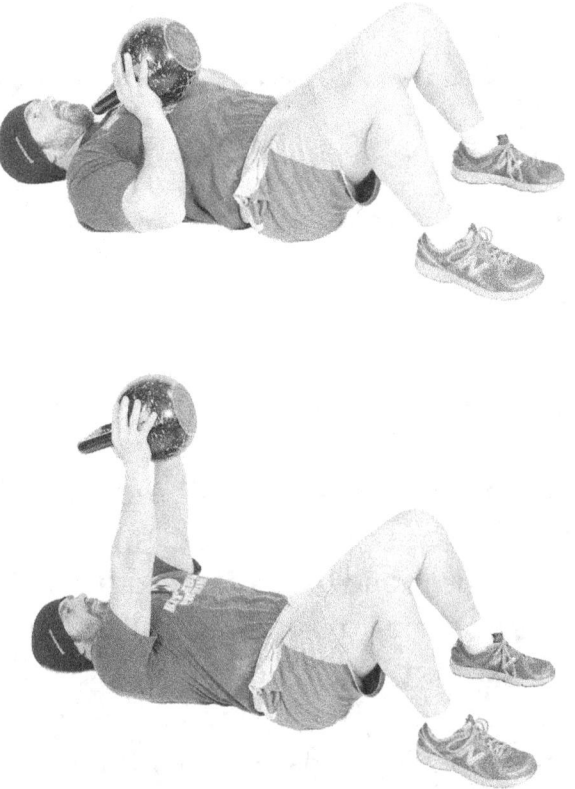

NOTE

If you are exercising on a hard surface, use a mat or some towels to cushion the floor.

SINGLE FLOOR PRESS

Lie on your back so that the kettlebell lines up with your midsection. Slide your hand through the handle with your palm up. Pull the kettlebell to your chest and turn your elbow out so that your upper arm is away from your body at roughly a 45-degree angle.

Keeping your knees bent and your feet flat on the floor, extend your free arm away from your body to help counter-balance the weight of the kettlebell on the other side. Take a deep breath then exhale forcefully and press the kettlebell until your arm is fully extended. Then slowly lower the kettlebell until your elbow gently touches the floor. Keeping the tension in your chest, shoulder, and triceps, press the weight back up for the next repetition.

By varying the position of the active arm you can emphasize different muscle groups with the Single Floor Press and other floor press variations. Keeping your elbow close to your body will emphasize the triceps. A wider elbow will emphasize the outer chest. To build in variety, you can switch your grip periodically. Experiment with these grip variations and decide which grip best suits your needs. In addition, all Floor Press variations can be performed with a pause in the bottom position to emphasize the development of the starting strength required to perform the movement. Simply hold the kettlebell(s) in the bottom position, keeping the muscles of the chest, shoulders and triceps tight, for a long pause before beginning the press.

SINGLE FLOOR PRESS: KEY POINTS

1. Lie on your back with your knees bent, so that the kettlebell is lined up with your abdomen.
2. Slide your hand through kettlebell handle with palm up.
3. Extend free arm away from body.
4. Pull kettlebell to chest and turn elbow out.
5. Take deep breath and press kettlebell to full extension.
6. Slowly lower kettlebell until elbow gently touches floor.
7. Pause briefly, keeping tension through chest, shoulder, and triceps.
8. Press back up.

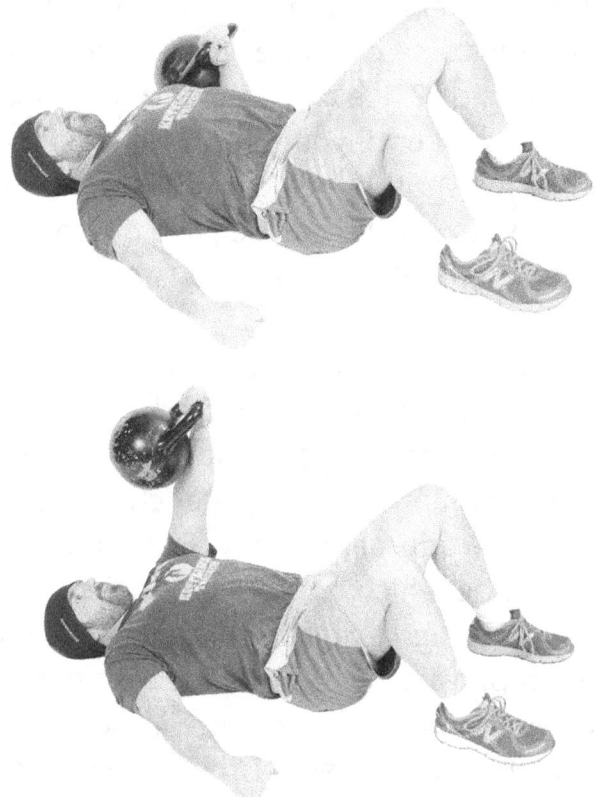

DOUBLE FLOOR PRESS

Set two kettlebells on the floor slightly wider than shoulder-width. Lie on your back between the kettlebells so that they are lined up with your midsection. Slide your hands through the handles with your palms up and pull the weights to your chest. As with the single floor press, turn your elbows out so that your arms are away from your body at an approximately a 45-degree angle. Keeping your knees bent and your feet flat on the floor, take a deep breath then exhale forcefully. As you exhale, press both kettlebells to a full extension and center them over your chest. Pause briefly, then slowly lower the kettlebells until your elbows gently touch the floor. Maintaining tension in your chest, shoulders, and triceps, pause briefly once again, then press up the kettlebells for the next repetition.

DOUBLE FLOOR PRESS: KEY POINTS

1. Set 2 kettlebells on floor slightly wider than shoulder-width.
2. Lie on your back between the kettlebells so the handles are lined up with your midsection.
3. Slide hands through handles, palms up.
4. Pull kettlebells to chest and turn elbows out.
5. Press to full extension over center of chest.
6. Pause at top, then lower slowly until elbows lightly touch floor.
7. Pause at bottom while keeping tension in chest, shoulders, and triceps.
8. Press up for next repetition.

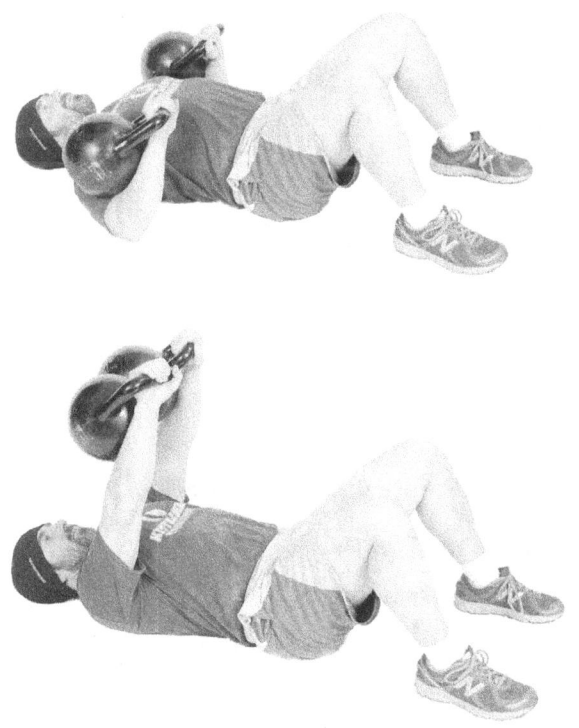

ALTERNATING (SEESAW) FLOOR PRESS

In this variation of the floor press, one of the kettlebells will be moving at all times. Set up as you would for a Double Press. Take a deep breath then press one kettlebell over your chest. As you lower the first kettlebell, begin to press the other kettlebell. Continue to alternate pressing the kettlebells in this fashion until your set is complete.

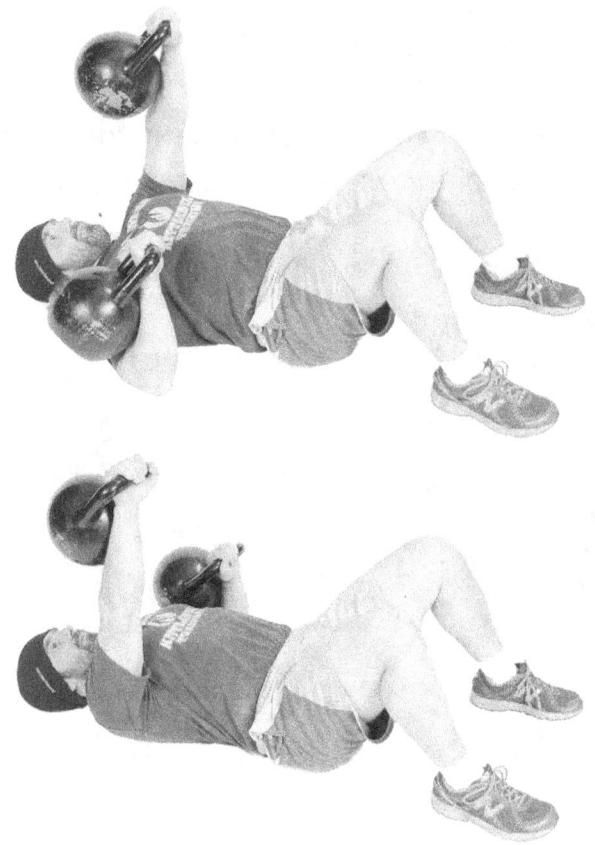

ALTERNATING (SEESAW) FLOOR PRESS: KEY POINTS

1. Set up as you would for a Double Press.
2. Press one kettlebell to full extension.
3. As you lower the first kettlebell, begin to press the second kettlebell.
4. Continue to alternate until set is complete.

ONE-STAYS-UP FLOOR PRESS

Here you will also alternate pressing the kettlebells, however, one of the kettlebells will be fully extended over your chest at all times. This exercise effectively works the small stabilizing muscles of the rotator cuff as well as the chest, triceps, and shoulders.

Set up as you would for any double floor press. Take a deep breath then press both kettlebells over your chest. Keeping one arm extended, bring the other kettlebell down until your elbow gently touches the floor. Press it back up and pause briefly with both kettlebells fully extended, then press the second ketllebell in the same fashion. Continue to alternate sides until your set is complete.

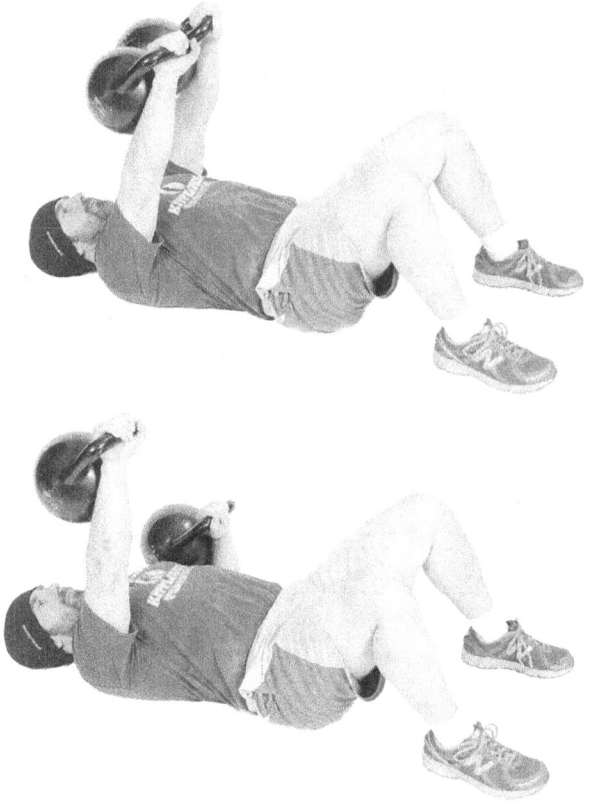

ONE-STAYS-UP FLOOR PRESS: KEY POINTS

1. Set up as you would for any Double Press.
2. Press both kettlebells to full extension.
3. Keeping one arm extended, lower the other kettlebell until elbow gently touches the floor.
4. Press kettlebell back up, pause; then lower the other kettlebell.
5. Continue to alternate in this fashion until set is complete.

NOTE

For variety or increased difficulty and abdominal development, Press Ups make great additions to any workout. The difference between a Floor Press and a Press Up is that when performing Press Ups, you actually flex the torso—sometimes moving both forward and diagonally—at the top of the movement, with your upper body rising off of the floor. Press Ups can be performed with the same variations as Floor Presses, such as single, double, two-handed, alternating, and one-stays-up.

To perform Press Ups, set up as you would for a floor press. For a Single Press Up, begin pressing one kettlebell to full extension so it is lined up with the middle of your chest. Brace your free arm against the floor, and as you press the kettlebell, rise off of the floor into a diagonal crunch. You will rise up onto the elbow of your free arm. Slowly lower your back, shoulders, and head; then bend your elbow until it gently touches the floor. Repeat the press and crunch with the opposite side. Continue to alternate sides until your set is complete.

CHAPTER 8
More Heavy Kettlebell Lifts

SIDE BEND (WINDMILL)

This exercise is great for developing strength, flexibility, and balance in your midsection. Snatch or clean-and-press a kettlebell overhead. Take a wide stance, wider than hip-width. Turn the foot of your free side so that it is perpendicular to the foot of your weighted side. Lower your free hand to the inside of your thigh and turn your palm up. Look up at the kettlebell then very slowly start to lean to your free side. Bend the knee of your free side as well then begin to lean forward slightly. Your goal should be to eventually be able to slide your free hand to the inside of your foot. When you have stretched as far as you are able, straighten back up to your starting position. Perform just a handful of repetitions before you switch to the other side. This is an exercise that takes great concentration and needs to be performed very slowly. I recommend repetition ranges of 3–5 per set.

SIDE BEND (WINDMILL): KEY POINTS

1. Snatch or Clean-and-Press kettlebell overhead.
2. Take wide stance.
3. Turn free foot until it is perpendicular to opposite foot.
4. Place free hand inside of thigh with palm up.
5. Look up at kettlebell then very slowly start to lean away from weight.
6. Bend free knee slightly then begin to lean forward while continuing to look at kettlebell.

7. Slide hand as low as you are able.
8. Slowly straighten up for next repetition.

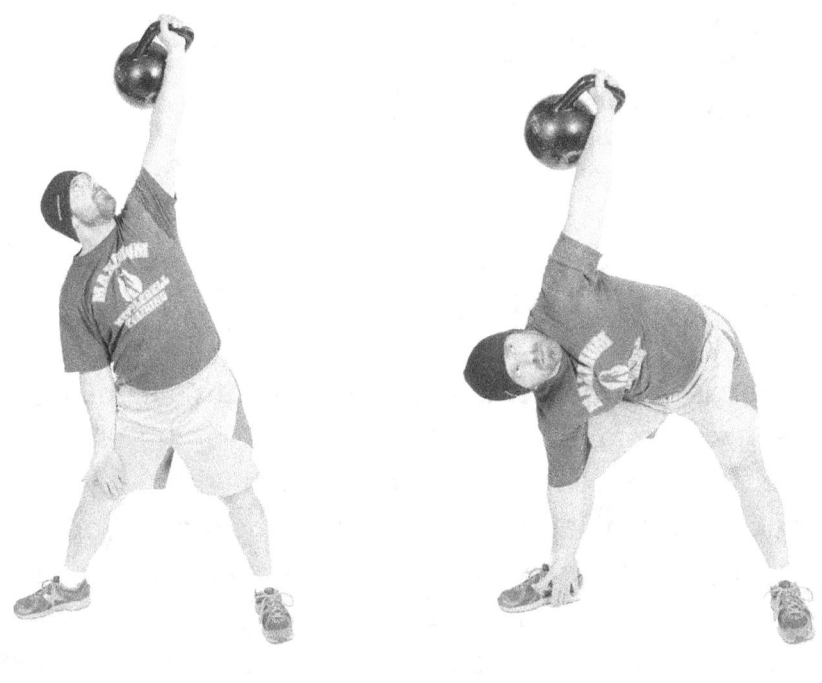

Squat Press

The Squat Press can be performed with either one or two kettle-bells. If using two, clean them to your shoulders. If using one, rest the kettlebell on your chest with the handle facing your body. Make sure to wrap your thumbs around the handle to secure the weight. Looking straight ahead, bend your knees as far as you are able. Your goal is to drop your hips lower than your knees. Then extend your knees and hips. When your legs and hips reach a fully erect position, continue the movement by pressing the kettlebell(s) overhead. Pause briefly then lower the kettlebell(s) back to a racked position on your chest or on the outside of your shoulders. As soon as the weight(s) makes contact with your chest or shoulders, drop down into the next repetition.

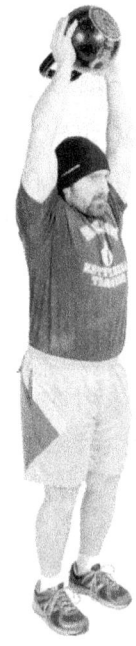
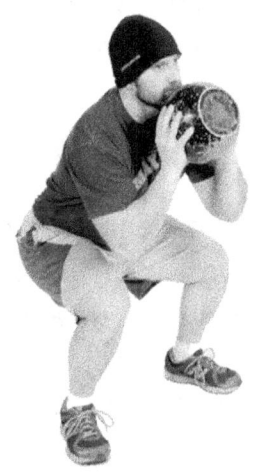

SQUAT PRESS: KEY POINTS

1. Position yourself with either one kettlebell on your chest or one on each shoulder in racked position.
2. Look straight ahead and bend knees then hips into a deep squat. Your goal is to drop your hips lower than your knees.
3. Press feet into floor and explode out of bottom position.
4. When you are standing erect, follow through into press.
5. Pause then lower kettlebell(s) back to a racked position.
6. As soon as the kettlebells make contact with your body, drop into next repetition.

SIDEWINDER (OFF CENTER HIGH PULL)

The Sidewinder is a variation of the High Pull that was discussed in an earlier chapter. It is a great exercise for grappling sports like wrestling, translating well to such moves as drilling pick-ups and double-leg takedowns. Otherwise, this variation is great for spicing up a stale routine.

Begin by setting up as you would for a High Pull. As you extend your knees and hips lean to the side, away from the kettlebell. At this point pull with your top arm, further bending your elbow. As you lower the weight, center your trunk once again. Explode out of the bottom position and repeat with the other side. Continue to alternate sides until your set is complete.

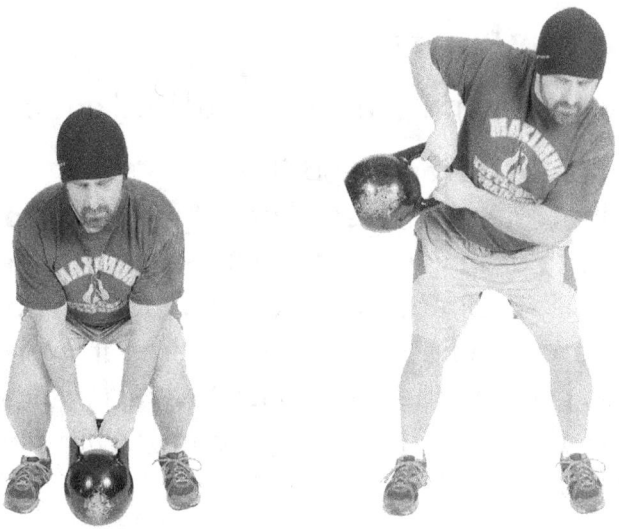

SIDEWINDER (OFF CENTER HIGH PULL): KEY POINTS

1. Set up as you would for a High Pull.
2. Extend knees and hip and begin pulling kettlebell toward chin.
3. Lean to one side, away from kettlebell.

4. Continue pulling with top elbow.
5. Center up as you lower weight.
6. Switch sides as you drive up for next repetition.

....

BENT PRESS

The Bent Press is a classic lift that was performed extensively by strength legends like Arthur Saxon, who in the 1920's could Bent-Press a barbell of well over 300 pounds with one hand. Though rarely practiced today, this old-school lift is great for developing strength, flexibility, and balance in your midsection, as well as pressing power in your arms and shoulders.

Begin by cleaning a kettlebell to a racked position, on the outside of your shoulder. Then take a rather wide stance, considerably greater that hip-width. Look at the kettlebell, then lean both forward and to your free side, as you would for a Side Bend. The knee of your free side should now be bent. Tense the musculature of your weighted side including the trapezius of the upper back as well as your abdominal and low back musculature. Take a deep breath then simultaneously press the weight up and drop your torso so that your elbow is now resting on the thigh of your free side. Essentially, you are both pressing the weight and dipping your body away from it. At this point the weight should be in a locked out position with your arm completely straight. Maintaining visual contact with the weight, straighten your torso until it is in an upright position. Then, lower the kettlebell back to a racked position on the outside of your shoulder and either prepare for the next repetition or switch sides. Since the Bent Press requires a considerable amount of concentration and core strength, keep your repetition ranges rather low. Sets of 3 to 5 repetitions work well.

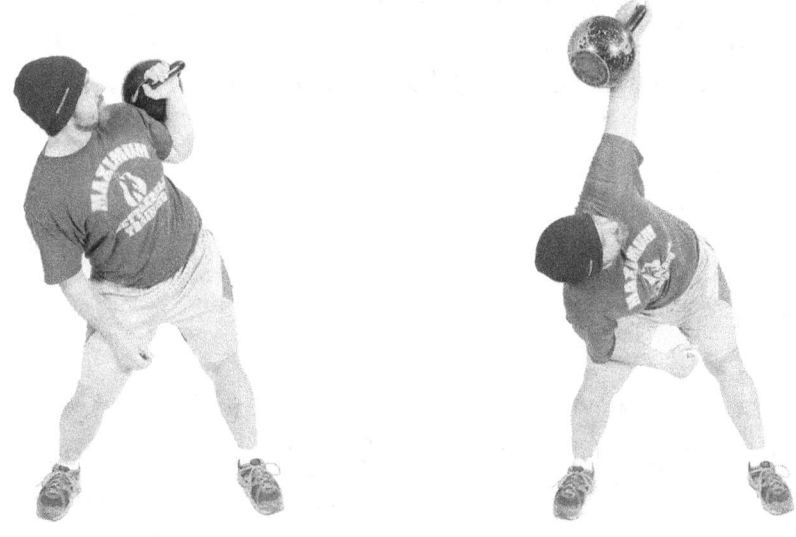

Bent Press: Key points

1. Clean the kettlebell to a racked position on the outside of your shoulder.
2. Widen your stance to greater than hip-width.
3. While maintaining visual contact with the kettlebell, tense the musculature of your core and upper back.
4. Take a deep breath then exhale and simultaneously lean forward and press away from the kettlebell until your arm is locked out and completely straight.
5. While maintaining visual contact with the kettlebell, straighten your torso.
6. Lower the kettlebell to a racked position on the outside of your shoulder.
7. Prepare for the next repetition or switch sides.

Note

When performing the Bent Press, the kettlebell should always be lined up with the center of your base of support. This is the point directly between your feet. To help keep this proper body alignment, your eyes should never leave the kettlebell.

TWO HANDS ANYHOW

The Two Hands Anyhow, another classic lift that was performed extensively by the strongmen of the late nineteenth and early twentieth centuries, demands the strength and flexibility of the Bent Press combined with an even greater need for balance and postural control.

Begin as you would for a Bent Press, by cleaning a kettlebell to a racked position, on the outside of your shoulder. Then take a rather wide stance, considerably greater that hip-width. Look up at the kettlebell, and then lean both forward and to your free side. The knee of your free side should now be bent. Tense the musculature of your weighted side including the trapezius of your upper back as well as your abdominal and low back musculature. Take a deep breath then simultaneously press the weight up and drop your torso so that your elbow is now resting on the thigh of your free side. Essentially, you are both pressing the weight and dipping your body away from it. At this point the weight should be in a locked out position with your arm completely straight. While bent over, you will then curl or lever a second kettlebell from the floor to a racked position, on the outside of your other shoulder.

Maintaining visual contact with the weight, straighten your torso until it is in an upright position. The first kettlebell should already be locked-out overhead, while the second kettlebell is still in the racked position. Next, press the second kettlebell overhead until it is locked out as well. Then, lower both kettlebells back to a racked position on the outside of your shoulders and then set them both down on the floor to prepare for the next repetition.

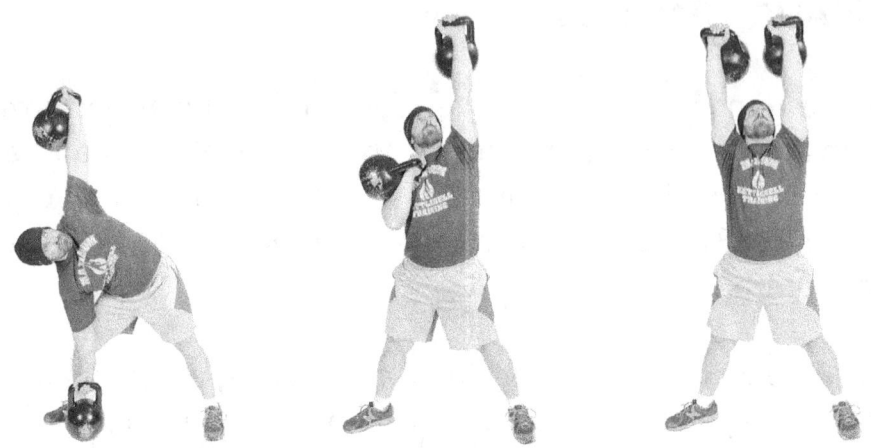

TWO HANDS ANYHOW: KEY POINTS

1. Clean the kettlebell to a racked position on the outside of your shoulder.
2. Widen your stance to greater than hip-width.
3. While maintaining visual contact with the kettlebell, tense the musculature of your core and upper back.
4. Take a deep breath then exhale and simultaneously lean forward and press away from the kettlebell until your arm is locked-out and completely straight.
5. Curl second kettlebell to a racked position on the outside of your other shoulder.
6. While maintaining visual contact with the kettlebell, straighten your torso.
7. Press the second kettlebell overhead to a locked-out position.
8. Lower both kettlebells back to a racked position on the outside of your shoulders.
9. Set both weights down on the floor.
10. Prepare for next repetition.

CHAPTER 9
My Favorite Non-Kettlebell Exercises

THICK BAR DEADLIFTS

Thick Bar Deadlifts became a staple for many strength enthusiasts after the appearance of Brooks Kubik's Dinosaur Training in 1996. I highly recommend this book, which describes strength training methods and tools from the past that will be a distant memory for some people and completely unknown to others. Typically, a thick bar would be 2 inches in diameter and 7 feet long, though shorter 48-inch bars can also been used. Incorporating thick bars, 2 inches or greater in diameter, will greatly improve your crushing and static grip strength, thus aiding your ability to lift kettlebells and other objects. The addition of thick bar training to your training regimen will also improve your overall strength for lifting odd objects due to the increased grip tension required in this type of training. This increased tension will force the body to innervate more motor units in the muscles of the hands and forearms, improving neuro-

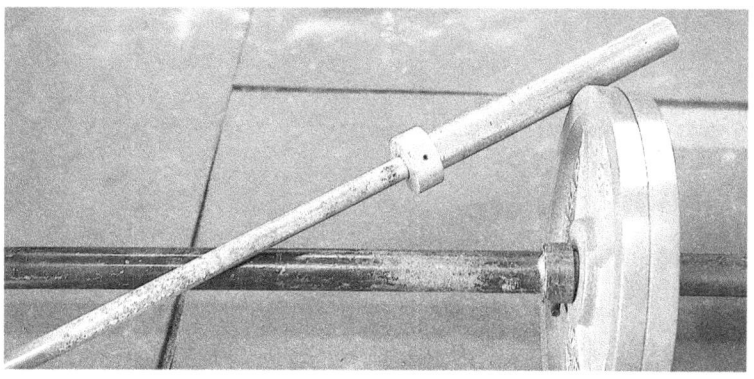

musclar efficiency, thus improving strength. By improving your grip and forearm strength you will also likely improve any pulling-type lift such as the clean, snatch, or deadlift.

My first Thick Bar was a gift from Canadian strongman John Hadzi, who attributed much of his grip and overall body strength to thick-bar work. Brooks Kubik's standard was that a strong man should be able to deadlift 300 pounds or more using a double prone (palms down) grip. This sounds simple, but for those of us with small hands it takes some work to achieve this. I often incorporate prone, thick-bar deadlifts every other week on my heavy day. I typically use a conventional (hands outside feet), hip-width stance, but these deadlifts work just as well for wide-stance, sumo style (hands inside feet) lifters. Thick-Bar Deadlifts also work well for deadlift assistance exercises such as Romanian Deadlifts and Stiff Leg Deadlifts.

I start with a moderate weight, performing triples and eventually switching to singles, and will keep adding weight until I hit a 1Repetition Maximum (1RM). (For those not familiar with this jargon, a repetition maximum is the maximum number of repetitions you can perform with a given load. For example, a 5 RM is the most weight you can use for 5 repetitions.) At this point I will stagger my grip, go back to triples, and work back up to a new 1RM. Thick-Bar Deadlifts can also be performed in a rack off of pins for maximal or near maximal weights, or standing on a block for a longer range of motion.

....

WEIGHTED CHIN-UPS

Old-fashioned chin-ups are often overlooked by strength enthusiasts, though they are making a comeback with the growing popularity of Crossfit and tactical-style workouts. The bottom line is that chin-ups, weighted or not, are hard for big men to do. Some time ago I was told a story about Mark Henry and John Brookfield. Henry, WWF star, powerlifter, and Olympian, once challenged grip-strength legend and Guinness record-holder Brookfield to a strength contest. As the story goes, they were in a weight gym and Mark, in good humor, said "Alright Brookfield, I challenge you to a lifting contest. You can pick anything in here, but none of that grip stuff." Though John had some of the strongest hands in history, was big by most standards, and had great overall body strength, he was

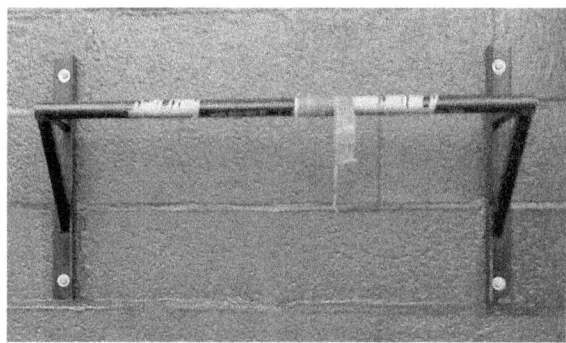

no match for Mark's massive 400+ pound body in a conventional head-to-head contest. Not only could Mark squat the equivalent in weight of a small truck, he could Olympic-lift with the best in the world. John, ever the thinker, paused and said, "Ok, how about chin-ups?" Mark rolled his eyes and said, "Shoot!" He knew John had him.

Why chin-ups? Why not stick with lat pulldowns or Hammer machine rows? I read an article in strength training journal *Milo* ages ago about a simple workout of dips, chin-ups, and squats. It was the author's opinion that a man should be able to perform at least 10 bodyweight chin-ups. Many tactical athletes are required to perform 20 or more in full tactical gear weighing up to 45 pounds. Personally, I prefer low-tech when it comes to equipment, training, and exercises. This is why chin-up variations appeal to me. In addition, I have found that weighted chin-ups work the lats and elbow flexors better than almost any other exercise and make great assistance exercises for kettlebell cleans and other pulls.

Perform weighted chin-ups on heavy days, after cleans or snatches. If you have neglected chip-ups, start with just your bodyweight and work up to 5 repetitions. Once you are able to perform sets of 5, begin adding weight using a dip belt, chain, rope, or other type of cord and increase weight in 5-pound increments. Making sure your form is perfect and you are not kicking, work up to a 1RM. Rotate prone, supine, and staggered grips with various widths each week or two on heavy days and stick to bodyweight on one power day at the beginning of the week.

Close-Grip Bench Press

I was fortunate enough in my early years to work with a coach who was a big proponent of close-grip bench presses. It is my humble opinion that this type of bench press is one of, if not THE, best triceps exercise. The close hand positioning lends itself to most major sports. Your chest, shoulders, and triceps have no choice but to work hard, as you are unable to use the leverage advantage of a wide grip. Famed powerlifting coach Louie Simmons swears by close-grip bench presses and has made them a staple for upper body work. You can perform these with weight only, or with the addition of bands, chains, hanging weights, or any combinations of these. I prefer to use a light, 10RM weight with bands for doubles and triples on Day 1 as an explosive assistance exercise to my overhead power work. I will also occasionally use them on my Day 3 heavy day and work up to a 1RM, though I only do this once every 3 or 4 weeks.

Whether you choose to bench flat, inclined, or declined, use a grip that is no wider than shoulder-width. Most lifters should have their index finger on the very edge of the knurling or just inside it. Make sure that you have a lift from a spotter or are using a rack with pins set at the appropriate height. The bar will be higher than it is when you use a wider grip. Lower the bar to the highest point of your chest or just below it and pull your elbows in slightly. Whether performing on your power day or your heavy, max-effort day, lift explosively throughout the range of motion.

BOX SQUATS

Certainly I am a tremendous fan of squats in general. Back squats, front squats, pauses, and lockouts. Few exercises have humbled me more than overhead squats. However, if I had to pick one squat style that would best complement kettlebell training, it would be the box squat. For those who are unfamiliar with this lift, the simple definition of box squats is using a back squat technique on a box or a low bench and pausing at the lowest point in the squatting movement, then explosively rising out of the bottom position. Though box heights vary, most lifters typically use one that will require them to squat below parallel, where the crease in their hip drops below the height of their knees. Occasionally, however, a higher box height might be warranted. For example, when an athlete wants to work on a particular range of motion, such as a lock-out. Regardless of position, this type of squatting develops great power that is highly beneficial for any athlete, but especially those in power and strength sports such as Olympic weight-lifting, powerlifting, kettlebell sport, and track and field. For a much more detailed explanation, I highly recommend the Westside Book of Methods, by Louie Simmons (2007).

Having done box squats on and off for years, I have determined that my kettlebell lifting is far better with them than without them. I prefer to keep the weight fairly light, around a 10RM, and perform doubles and triples, usually for 6 sets. Weight alone on a straight bar works well if the lift is properly performed, but I find that the addition of bands provides a little more benefit. Decades ago, when I first began box squatting, I used too much weight and would either rock forward coming off the bench or actually bounce off a high bench. This lack of technique is not only unsafe, but also unproductive. I recommend the Westside style, which calls for a low box, and pausing at the bottom of the movement then coming straight up. (I use an 11 inch milk crate. I'm short, so don't judge me!) Powerlifters may want to use a wide stance, but since we are discussing the box squat as an assistance lift for kettlebell training, I would recommend a hip-width stance, driving your feet into the floor like you are trying to jump. I have found that this variation of box squatting helps develop the explosive leg drive that is essential for heavy cleans and pulls.

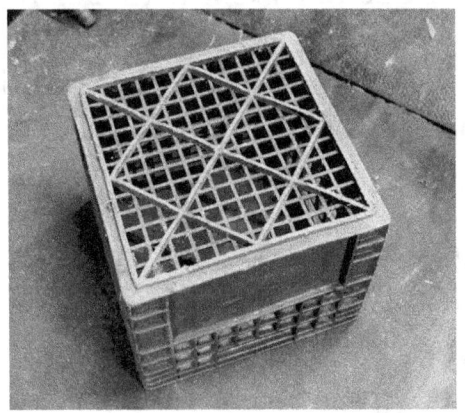

CHAPTER 10
Putting It All Together

PROGRAM DESIGN

Over the years I have come to believe that the surest way to screw up a good strength training program is to overcomplicate it. Simple programs, when performed with enough intensity, volume, variety, and proper recovery, can produce great results. What I hope to accomplish in this chapter is to map out a step-by-step plan for developing maximal strength and power by using kettlebells as the main training implement. This program will also include some optional exercises using non-kettlebell strength training equipment that is readily available to most lifters. I have organized this program in a fashion that I have personally found to be the most beneficial through my many years of research, trial, and error.

I prefer a 4-day split routine, with Days 1 and 2 dedicated to power training and Days 3 and 4 dedicated to maximal strength. It is worth noting that when I competed in powerlifting, I used a program very different than what I describe here and more closely resembled a Linear Model of Periodization. I trained with heavy weights the majority of the time, with intervals of lighter, higher volume work. As a powerlifting meet grew near, I would gradually taper my assistance work. I routinely overtrained, however. It was only after I retired from powerlifting that I began to explore changing the speed of movement as one of my variables. I guess learning late is better than never. What I learned is to train hard and make gains, but to avoid overtraining. It only took me three decades and two college degrees to learn this. One addition I made to my training, however, was to add more variety to my heavy days. After just a few short weeks, I found that I could once again increase any of the main lifts on which I had been stalling. In fact, for some lifts I was able to improve weight for the first time in years. Though I had used box squats in the past, I was re-motivated to try them as an assistance exercise for my kettlebell work. They turned out to be a great addition to my program. For me, they are best employed after my kettlebell work on Day 2 of my program.

The following are sample workouts that closely resemble my own. These are intended to give you an idea where to begin in your own program design.

POWER DAYS

As I previously mentioned, I prefer to make days 1 and 2 of a four day split routine my power days. Since the focus of this book is the development of strength and power using kettlebells as the main training implement, we will use basic kettlebell exercises as the foundation of our training program. Because the Single Snatch does not come easy to me, I prefer to make it my primary exercise on Day 1. You may, however, focus on any major kettlebell power movement on Day 1, such as the Clean, Double Clean, or Double Snatch. I typically center Day 2 around the Single Clean and Press, in part because I am very confident with my Clean and Press, and in part because I feel that the combination of Cleans and Presses is one of the most practical strength combinations in existence. Other than the deadlift, few exercises have greater benefit in work and sport than the Clean and Press.

Regarding training variables on Power Days, I have found that due to the unilateral nature of many kettlebell exercises, traditional set, repetition, and intensity schemes vary somewhat from barbell training and the Olympic lifts. For single-sided exercises, I have found that four to six sets each side of one to three repetitions work well, as you might expect. If I perform more than four to six sets per side, fatigue begins to interfere with my technique. If you choose exercises that require two kettlebells, such as Double Snatches, for your foundational exercises, I recommend performing six to ten sets total. Assistance exercises must be practical and contribute to the progress of my foundational lifts. I find exercises such as High Pulls, Clean variations, Thick-Bar Deadlifts, Box Squats, Overhead Presses, and Close Grip Barbell Bench Presses extremely beneficial. I typically choose four to six assistance exercises to use for a three- to six-week period on Power Days. I usually perform these exercises for three to six repetitions, for three to six sets, and with a starting load equal to approximately 60% of my 1 repetition maximum (RM) or a weight that I can use for ten to twelve repetitions. I gradually increase weight over time. This next point is critical: Each repetition on the Power Days must be performed as explosively as safety allows. Training slowly with a light weight for few repetitions will provide little benefit to power development, therefore you must attack every repetition. I have found that one- to two-minute rest breaks work well for this type of training, though I personally rarely go beyond one-minute breaks. If you need more rest in the beginning, take it, though over time you should try to decrease the length of your breaks between sets.

MAXIMUM STRENGTH DAYS

Maximum strength days are a critical part of this type of program. Ultimately, you must lift heavy at some point to gain strength, but constantly training heavy will lead to overtraining. This sounds like common sense but the problem is more complicated on closer examination. Block training—working in phases dedicated to one training attribute, such as strength—can work well, but only for a short period before overtraining and/or injury sets in. Furthermore, it is easy to lose other training attributes such as power or muscular endurance when training exclusively one attribute. I have found that I can only train with near maximal weights for approximately three weeks before feeling negative effects. Even alternating heavy and light blocks, my results tend to be limited. Conversely, by training with reasonably light weights lifted in an explosive manner combined with near-maximal and maximal weights—which is to say a combination of Power Days and Maximal Strength Days—I realize a much better outcome. That said, I personally have found that performing the exact same heavy lifts on subsequent Maximum Strength Days leads to limited gains and moderate staleness. More recently, and largely due to some excellent advice I received, I have been rotating three to six main lifts on my Max Strength Days and have been realizing significantly better progress. I still max out my key lifts—Single Snatch and Single Clean and Press—but only every six weeks or so. My other Maximum Strength Days are focused on big movements that will contribute to my Snatches and Cleans. These other lifts may include Double Kettlebell Snatches, Barbell Squats and deadlifts, Barbell Snatches and Cleans, Stone lifting, Thick Bar work, Sandbag training, Power Rack partial squats and pulls, and so on.

Maximum Strength Days work best for me later in the week, but I suggest experimenting to see what works best for you. These days need to contribute to your overall goals, so exercise selection is critical to your success. For my own program I usually reserve one day for heavy ballistic work and/or leg work and one day for heavy pressing work. I have found over the years that my presses usually go down if performed after a heavy whole-body or leg day, so I prefer to perform my heavy presses on day three of a four-day split routine. Since I am working on improving my Single Overhead Press, I will rotate movements such as Barbell Bench Presses of close, medium and wide grips, Overhead Barbell Presses, Power Rack Overhead Barbell Lockouts, Single Overhead Dumbbell Presses, and other heavy pressing movements that I have found help me to increase my Single Overhead Kettlebell Press.

As with Power Days, assistance work for Maximum Strength Days typically consists of a handful of exercises that I find to be of value and that will contribute the most to my overall goals of improving my Single Snatch and Single Clean and Press. Personal favorites include Maximum Box Squats with bands, Overhand Thick Bar Deadlifts, Kettlebell Single and Double Outside Cleans, Double Snatches, and other similar exercises.

THREE-DAY PROGRAM SAMPLE

When designing a program with three lift days in a one-week microcycle, I would recommend using two power days, with one max strength day in between. An alternative for only the most advanced lifters might be to alternate power days with max strength days with an ABA format one week and BAB format the next, however, I have found that I cannot perform this type of routine indefinitely. Even though volume is relatively low, my back simply cannot recover from two maximal strength days in one week for more than a few weeks since the muscle groups used for many exercises overlap.

DAY 1

- Kettlebell Overhead Push Press with light bands for 6 sets of 3 repetitions (6x3) each side at 60% 1RM.
- Kettlebell Snatch or Clean for 6x2 with 10RM
- Close-Grip (shoulder-width) Bench Press with bands, 6x2 with 10RM
- Kettlebell Single Outside Clean 6x2 with 10RM
- Box Squats with bands 10RM, 6 sets of 2 with 10RM
- Kettlebell One-Handed High Pull 3x6 with 6-8RM

DAY 2

- Kettlebell Floor Press, relax and pause at bottom of every rep. Begin with triples, work up to best single.
- Kettlebell Swings, 2 hands or 1 hand. Begin with triples, work up to best single.
- Kettlebell Single Jerks, 6x3 each, work up to 3RM
- Weighted chin-ups 3x6 with 6-8RM
- Kettlebell Double High Pull 3x6 with 6-8RM
- Thick-Bar deadlift with overhand grip. Begin with triples, work up to best single.

DAY 3 (OPTIONAL VARIETY)

- Kettlebell Push Press, 10 RM weight, 6x3 each side
- Kettlebell Double Snatch, 10 RM weight, 10x2
- Low-incline kettlebell or dumbbell presses 3x6 with 6-8RM
- Kettlebell Alternating Cleans for speed 3x8 with 8-10RM
- Kettlebell Single Rows 4x10 each with 10-12RM
- Stiff-Leg deadlift 2x12 with 12-15RM

FOUR-DAY PROGRAM SAMPLE

DAY 1

- Kettlebell Overhead Push Press with light band 6x3 each side with 10RM
- Close-Grip (shoulder-width) Bench Press with bands 6x3 with 10RM
- Low-incline dumbbell bench press 3x6 with 6-8RM
- Lying barbell triceps extensions, 3x10 with 10-12RM
- Prone-grip body-weight chin-ups (performed with bottom pause and explosive upward movement) 3x6 with 6-8RM
- Weighted supine-grip chin-ups, 3x6 with 6-8RM
- EZ bar pullovers, 3x12 with 12-15RM

DAY 2

- Kettlebell Snatch, 6x2 each side with 10RM
- Kettlebell Outside Single Clean 6x2 with 10RM
- Box squats with bands, 6x2 with10RM
- Kettlebell One-Handed High Pull 3x6 with 6-8RM
- Romanian deadlift 3x6 with 6-8RM

DAY 3

- Standing barbell push press. Pause bottom position. Begin with triples, work up to best single.
- Barbell floor press, relax and pause at bottom of every rep. Begin with triples, work up to best single.
- Weighted dips, 3x6 with 6-8RM
- Weighted chin-ups to face, 3x6 with 6-8RM
- Kettlebell Bent-over Single Row, 3x6 with 6-8RM
- Barbell power shrugs, 3x6 with 6-8RM
- Alternating dumbbell curls 3x10 with 10-12RM

DAY 4

- Barbell high pull. Begin by performing triples and work up to best single.
- Kettlebell Swings. Begin with 1 hand and perform triples and work up to best single. Switch to 2 hands and perform triples and, once again, work up to best single. Use dumbbells or odd implements as necessary to increase weight.
- Overhand grip thick-bar deadlifts with bands. Begin with triples and work up to best single. Then, switch to a staggered grip and perform triples and, once again, work up to best single.
- Stiff leg barbell deadlifts 2x15

....

BONUS WORKOUTS

In addition to my main regularly scheduled training sessions, I like to incorporate 1–4 additional mini-sessions each week. I call these "bonus" workouts or "dessert" workouts, since my regular sessions would be the main course. Each bonus workout lasts approximately 20–30 minutes and usually consists of 1–4 exercises. I perform this type of workout out of necessity since I might not have time or energy to do it during my regular workouts. Bonus workouts may also be performed for a variety of other reasons. They might consist of work that is incompatible with your regular power or strength sessions, such as high intensity interval work. They may also be exercises or specialty work that you simply do not have time for in your sessions such as core or grip specialization. Or they may consist of some sort of rehabilitation work such as rotator cuff exercises, joint rehabilitation, or postural alignment. Whatever your reason, brief, specialty workouts can be a worthwhile addition to your main training sessions. I usually have time for 1 or 2 extra sessions per week, though I strive for 4. My bonus sessions usually consist of sled work, stone lifting, and/or mace work. Depending upon the time of year, I also try to incorporate some high repetition kettlebell exercises such as Single Snatches or Clean and Press combinations. The following are a few of my favorite bonus workouts. They are both fun and beneficial.

MACE / HAMMER SWINGS, CHOPS & TWISTS

Strength training enthusiasts have long been attracted to heavy hammers, axes, and clubs. There is simply something primal about swinging a weapon overhead, a martial art of ages past that has become a fixture of modern strength and conditioning. Strength training always seems to come back to the basics.

Recently, the resurgence of hammer training can be traced largely to the popularity of a mid-twentieth-century wrestler who went by the ring name of Karl Gotch. Well into his later years, Gotch could

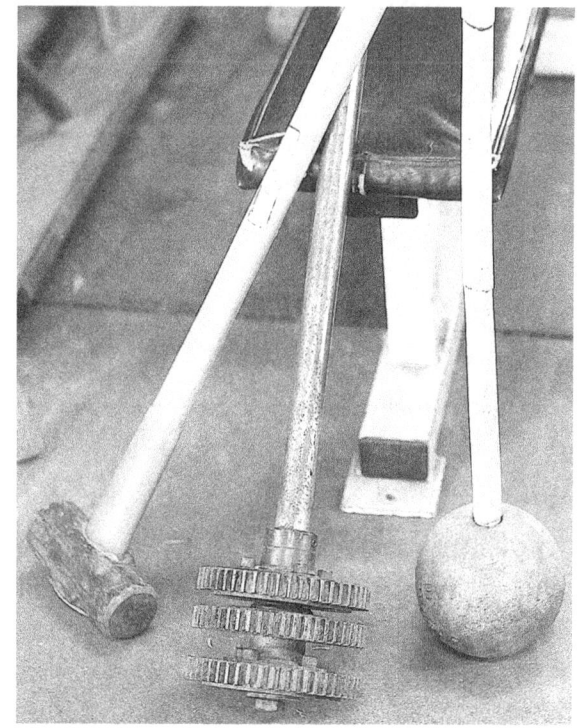

swing a heavy mace overhead for what seemed like forever. Maces and hammers continue to be a popular way for modern martial artists to gain the type of whole body strength that conventional gym training seems to miss.

After fooling around with light hammers for a while, I began working with a relatively heavy hammer. The challenge of hammer training, however, depends not only on the weight but also the length of the handle (or lever arm), hand placement, weight distribution, and overall exercise technique. My first custom hammer was made out of the gears of an old printing press and has the look of a medieval weapon. It is 44 inches long and weighs 35 pounds, though I have seen hammers as heavy as 60 pounds. Regardless of how heavy you start, make an effort to read up on basic mace and hammer swinging technique.

When most people think of training with hammers, they picture themselves hitting a tractor tire sledge-hammer style. While this certainly can be a valuable exercise, you have many more options with this great training implement and you are only limited by your imagination. I frequently perform overhead, mace-style swings either as part of a warm up or as part of a mini core/abdominal workout. Other great hammer movements include standing twists, diagonal swings, one-handed overhead swings with lighter hammers, various levering exercises... the list goes on.

Since you may not have access to a set of heavy hammers that increase in small weight increments, it is necessary to be creative to build progression into your training program. There are several straight-forward ways of making hammer lifting more challenging. You can alter the position of your hands relative to each other or relative to the length of the lever, you can change the distance between the handle and your body, and you can simply change the exercise.

I have found professional trainer and unconventional strength guru Rik Brown to be a wealth of knowledge. Rik has made a name for himself in strength and conditioning by developing expertise in mace and hammer training in addition to kettlebells. Sadly for me, he makes the hammers I swing look like swizzle sticks on an umbrella drink. A big man at six feet, seven inches, and 260 pounds, Rik has developed tremendous torque and power and a brutally strong grip

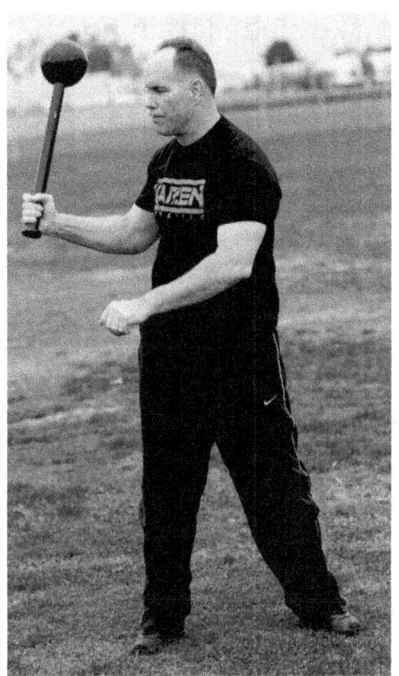

by swinging maces of various sizes. In the picture at left, Rik demonstrates the finer points of one-handed mace work. Rik encourages mace practitioners to swing for time instead of repetitions. A timer can be a great way to manipulate work/rest ratios rather than just adding weight or repetitions. Rik also suggests stopping your set when your technique begins to break down. This is especially important for older strength enthusiasts, myself included. Form comes first! (For more information on Rik Brown, see libertystregnthtraining.com.)

STONE LIFTING AND THROWING

There is something that draws me to stone lifting, maybe its primitiveness or fundamentality. I also like the way it pushes lifters out of their comfort zones, forcing them to twist, turn, and adjust to an oddly shaped object that has been around since the Earth was born. Whatever your reason for lifting stones, this type of training has undeniable value, and it is very compatible with kettlebell training. World's Strongest Man finalist Jesse Marunde trained with heavy kettlebells to enhance his stone lifting and said not only that he decreased his stone-lifting times, but also that he was able to lift heavier stones. Canadian strongman John Hadzi was known to lift, push, and pull tremendous stone loads in conjunction with heavy kettlebell Cleans, Presses, and Flips. Stone lifting gave John a kind of brute strength seldom seen in men of any size, let alone a man of 260 pounds, which is considered little in John's circles. John often used stones to build low back and crushing grip strength. In fact, he was so proficient in combining his stone and kettlebell training, that he was able to perform Kettlebell One-Handed Forward Flips with a 180+ pound kettlebell. This involves yanking a kettlebell of solid iron

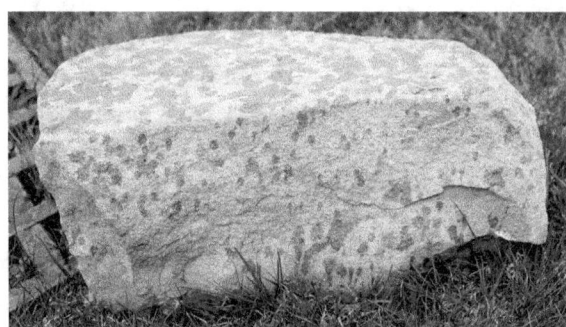

the size of a large globe off the ground with one hand to eye level, pushing the handle forward with enough force to rotate the kettlebell mid-air, grabbing the handle with the same hand, then lowering the weight to the ground under control. If that doesn't take whole body strength, I am not sure what does. The only other men to even come close to such a feat were Herman Goerner, a 315-pound man (considered giant in the 1940's) and grip-strength legend John Brookfield, the first kettlebell practitioner in modern times to flip turn a 145-pound kettlebell. What was their secret? All of these men trained on a regular basis with basic, crude implements including stones, hammers, and kettlebells.

I once dedicated an entire summer to heavy stone lifting and kettlebell basics. This turned out to be time well spent. My posterior chain musculature was never stronger. I was able to break all of my personal kettlebell records and also became quite proficient at stone lifting by focusing on shouldering large, oddly shaped mountain stones.

Stone putting and throwing are also great kettlebell assistance exercises. They allow the lifter to explode throughout the entire range of motion, something that doesn't happen in traditional kettlebell training alone. When performing Snatches and Cleans, the racking motion forces the lifter to slow the kettlebell; otherwise, the motion of the weight continues, likely resulting in injury. If, however, you are fortunate enough to have access to an outdoor training space, you can use small stones of various weights to enhance your kettlebell training with throws. Two-handed overhead throws are a great assistance exercise for Single and Double Snatches, because you can accelerate through the entire range. In addition, throwing stones shot-put style, by pressing off the shoulder and following through, is great for building strength to press one or two kettlebells off the shoulders for a max-effort Clean and Press. So, sticks and stones may break bones, but lifting them properly builds a stronger body.

SANDBAGS

Sandbags can be utilized in much the same way as stones. They can be cleaned, pressed, shouldered, and squatted. Two key differences are, however, that the weight in sandbags can shift, forcing lifters to constantly adjust their techniques. In addition, depending on the type of sandbag used and its weight, the sandbag cloth can sometimes be gripped, developing finger strength and allowing for exercises like Cleans and Snatches. I prefer old-fashioned Army duffles filled with sand for this type of training. They are washable and very durable, usually lasting quite a long time. Some newer sandbags, made specifically for strength and conditioning, have handles. Personally I think these detract from gains in grip strength and otherwise poses less of a challenge.

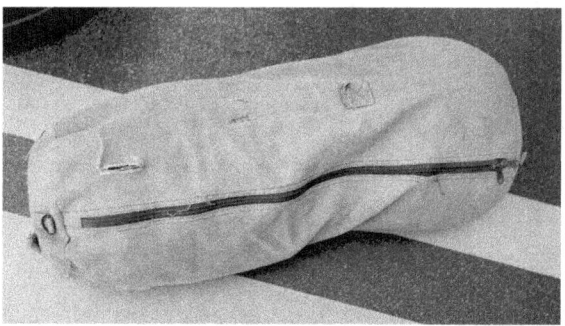

WHEELBARROWS, SLEDS & OTHER ODD OBJECTS

Most of us have engaged in pushing and pulling wheelbarrows, sleds, and other odd objects all of our lives for reasons other than strength training. Wrestling with a heavy wheelbarrow loaded with gravel around a yard or construction site or pushing a car out of a snow bank are the types of activities that jack the heart rate and develop whole-body strength like few other activities can. A college 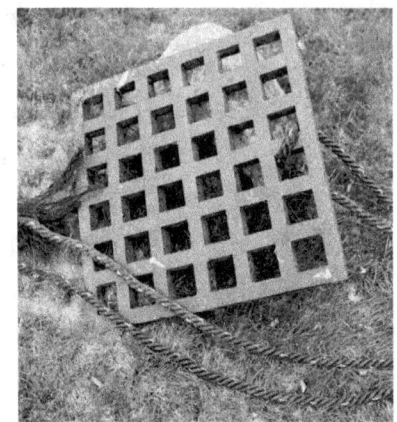 friend of mine with tremendous overall strength works a gazillion hours a week for a construction company. In order to get a workout in, he has to get it in at work. He will routinely load a wheelbarrow up to eye level with bags of cement and race up hills and over ruts at whichever job site he happens to be currently working. When possible, he will move materials manually, even though a forklift might be available. The bottom line is that he never misses an opportunity to build strength.

Another training partner of mine used to have his son, a 138-pound judo champion, load a wheelbarrow with 400 pounds of weight and wrestle it up and down the hills of their neighborhood. This type of training, along with mastery of core kettlebell exercises, allowed this young man to defeat competitors who were much larger and had decades more experience. They simply could not match his speed or strength.

Training sleds, another great training tool, have gained popularity in the last decade or so. A training sled usually consists of a flat peice of metal with a post for adding weight plates or a pair of rails made of round metal piping with crossbars and upright tubing for the addition of weight. Chains or ropes are then attached to the sled to allow the lifter to pull it. Some sleds also have grips that allowing for pushing as well as pulling. Though early sleds were usually home made implements, manufactured weight sleds eventually became available for purchase. If you

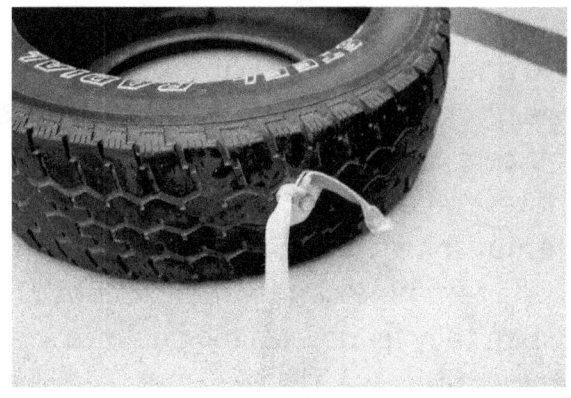

don't want to spring the cash for a new sled, it is not difficult to make your own. I tied a rope around an old 150-pound sewer grate and use it to perform various sprints with arms extended, both forward and backward, as wells as high pulls for my short specialty workouts or at the end of a session. This type of work can be performed for speed, conditioning, or anything else you need. You are only limited by your imagination. Another method of sled building comes from Jerry Shreck, head strength coach at Bucknell University. Coach Shreck takes a regular car tire and cuts a ring in the side wide enough to fit 45-pound weight plates. He attaches two eye bolts with washers to the tire so that chains or ropes may be attached. He then inserts a board or piece of plywood into the tire to help secure the weight plates or anything else he puts in it. He then places weight plates and/or other heavy objects in the tire. Multiple tires may be towed or attached to one another if additional weight is needed.

John Hadzi, the Canadian strongman and trainer, will load up a reinforced cart with 800 pounds worth of stones, sandbags, and kettlebells and run up the hills in his Toronto neighborhood. Though this might be quite a sight for the average person, anyone with an ounce of strength training knowledge will recognize it as a tremendous feat, let alone a regular workout. The police once stopped John because they believed the cart might contain body parts wrapped in duffel bags! When their suspicions were allayed, they asked John what he could possibly be doing. John responded, "I'm working out, of course." The officers didn't believe him and said, "You're lying. No one can lift this." Without another word, John yanked one of the weight filled bags out of the cart and effortlessly shouldered it. The officers were in awe! The police never bothered him again. A quick note: You may want to secure your kettlebells should you ever attempt John's workout. If the cart or wheelbarrow tips over, kettlebells resemble cannon balls in both look and destructive potential when they fly down a hill and into a parked car. Don't ask me how I know this!

AFTERWORD
Kettlebells and Strength Training:
Now More Than Ever!

I have always admired strength. When I was a kid growing up in the northeast, strength training was the only thing that got me through those long, dark winters. I remember getting up at 3:30 a.m. to meet my coach at the gym by 4. No, this isn't where I say that I walked twenty miles up hill both ways to get there, but the truth is that the gym was in the bottom of a warehouse with no heat. In the middle of winter it took a special amount of determination and discipline to get out of bed to workout. Though this was twenty years before the return of kettlebell training, I was learning that the best results came from simple, time-tested equipment and straight-forward training.

Lifting weights was all I thought about then (except for girls), much to the detriment of my math grades. When I wasn't working out, I was developing programs for myself and others. They would consist of numerous sets of squats, deadlifts, presses, and any other big lifts I could think of that might give me the sort of strength and muscular thickness that my heroes had. I remember watching the enormous powerlifter Mike Hall on TV next to former LA Raider Lyle Alzado. At a bodyweight of 400 pounds, Hall simply dwarfed Alzado. As a demonstration of his strength and muscular endurance, Hall began bench-pressing 315 pounds. The show went on commercial break and came back several minutes later and Hall was still pressing the weight for reps.

Though my body and my lifestyle have changed over the years, with long commutes and crazy family and work schedules, I love strength training now more than ever. After my powerlifting days, I was at a loss for what direction to take my training. I still wanted to lift heavy weights and objects, but I also sought a broader spectrum of training outcomes. I now had to work for the athleticism I took for granted earlier in my life. I now had to build muscular endurance and agility into my program, because they simply were going away with age.

It was during this transition in my personal strength and conditioning that I was introduced to kettlebell training. Though I was aware of kettlebells, their value was lost on me. I simply did not know enough about them. At this time they had not gained much popularity in modern training systems and most lifters considered them little more than weird-looking iron balls that old timers used. Heavy kettlebells were not yet available and the big men that used the lighter ones swore they ruined their lifts.

I was reluctant to work with them at first, but a friend and mentor insisted they would give me the combination of power, strength, agility, and stamina I so desperately sought. I am now eternally grateful to this friend and glad that I listened. Since that time I have dedicated my professional career to finding the best training implements and methodologies for producing specific strength and conditioning results. In all of my research, trial, and error, I can honestly say that kettlebells, whether alone or in combination with other implements, are one of the greatest tools—if not *the* greatest tool—for developing strength and power. They are the perfect middle ground between the Olympic lifts and the big three power lifts. They give the lifter whole-body power for pick-ups, pulls, twists, and throws. They will help you punch harder, jump higher, and run faster. The versatility of kettlebells is unparalleled, as there is almost no exercise or training attribute in existence where they will not be of great benefit.

If it is strength and power you seek, kettlebells will be a great addition to your training regimen, whether used exclusively or in conjunction with barbells, dumbbells, stones, sandbags, or some other basic training tools. They will enhance everything from the way you grip to the way you stand. Regular, properly organized, kettlebell training will give you the constant feeling that you are physically powerful. You will *feel* stronger. It is the type of whole-body work strength that comes into play regardless of where you are. Whether you are on the playing field, in the gym, or moving an odd object, kettlebell training will make it easier.

I hope you enjoyed reading this book as much as I have enjoyed writing it. I wish you well in your strength and conditioning endeavors.

Yours in strength and health,

Dave Bellomo

www.ingramcontent.com/pod-product-compliance
Lightning Source LLC
Chambersburg PA
CBHW081837280526
45789CB00007B/2479